PANCREATIC CANCER

A Patient & His Doctor Balance Hope & Truth

A JOHNS HOPKINS PRESS HEALTH BOOK

PANCREATIC CANCER

A Patient & His Doctor Balance Hope & Truth

Michael J. Lippe *and* Dung T. Le, M.D.

THE JOHNS HOPKINS UNIVERSITY PRESS

Baltimore

Note to the Reader. One of the authors of *Pancreatic Cancer: A Patient and His Doctor Balance Hope and Truth* is a person who has pancreatic cancer, and the book, in part, is a first-person account of his experience. The other author is a physician who is providing his medical care. This book is intended to acquaint readers with some of the emotions and practical issues that may be involved in the experience of having pancreatic cancer, as well as with some of the expertise and thoughts involved in making decisions when providing medical care to someone who has pancreatic cancer. The book is not meant to substitute for medical care of people with pancreatic cancer, and medical treatment should not be based solely on its contents. Instead, treatment must be developed in a dialogue between the individual and his or her physician. This book is a model of one dialogue and has been written to enhance other dialogues.

Drug dosage: The author and publisher have made reasonable efforts to determine that the selection and dosage of drugs discussed in this text conform to the practices of the general medical community at the time of publication. The medications described do not necessarily have specific approval by the U.S. Food and Drug Administration for use in the diseases and dosages for which they are recommended. In view of ongoing research, changes in governmental regulations, and the constant flow of information relating to drug therapy and drug reactions, the reader is urged to check the package insert of each drug for any change in indications and dosage and for warnings and precautions. This is particularly important when the recommended agent is a new and/or infrequently used drug.

© 2011 The Johns Hopkins University Press
All rights reserved. Published 2011
Printed in the United States of America on acid-free paper
2 4 6 8 9 7 5 3 1

The Johns Hopkins University Press
2715 North Charles Street
Baltimore, Maryland 21218-4363
www.press.jhu.edu

Library of Congress Cataloging-in-Publication Data
Lippe, Michael J.
Pancreatic cancer : a patient and his doctor balance hope and truth /
Michael J. Lippe and Dung T. Le.
p. cm.
Includes bibliographical references and index.
ISBN-13: 978-1-4214-0061-7 (hardcover : alk. paper)
ISBN-10: 1-4214-0061-8 (hardcover : alk. paper)
ISBN-13: 978-1-4214-0062-4 (pbk. : alk. paper)
ISBN-10: 1-4214-0062-6 (pbk. : alk. paper)
1. Lippe, Michael J.—Health. 2. Pancreas—Cancer—Popular works.
I. Le, Dung T. II. Title.
RC280.P25L5 2011
616.99'437—dc22   2010042497

A catalog record for this book is available from the British Library.

Illustrations on pages 14, 15, 42, 107, and 111 are by Jacqueline Schaffer.

Special discounts are available for bulk purchases of this book. For more information, please contact Special Sales at 410-516-6936 or specialsales@press.jhu.edu.

The Johns Hopkins University Press uses environmentally friendly book materials, including recycled text paper that is composed of at least 30 percent post-consumer waste, whenever possible. All of our book papers are acid-free, and our jackets and covers are printed on paper with recycled content.

CONTENTS

Postscript 147

Contents   vii

PREFACE

The roots of our journey, and this book, lie in the collaboration and the dialogue that we have had over the past several years. It is not a journey that either of us would have chosen, had we been given a choice. As with so many other things in life, we were not asked.

In some sense, there was also little choice in whether or not to write about what was happening. The idea of writing about this experience and about the broader subject of pancreatic cancer from the patient's and the physician's perspectives came to us in the middle of 2009. Like so much of our dialogue, this conversation started with an e-mail, this one from Michael to Dung, a simple question: Would you like to collaborate on writing a book?

We recognize that our collaboration is unusual. It is not completely unheard of, but it is unusual. Documenting the unusual seems to both of us to be important for many reasons. Foremost among these is the belief that telling one patient's story from his perspective and combining it with a detailed account of what is taking place medically can help the tens of thousands of people who are diagnosed with pancreatic cancer each year.

A diagnosis of pancreatic cancer, indeed any cancer that is potentially fatal in a short period of time, is a paralyzing event. Trying to demystify what is going on, and to make the unknown a little less forbidding, became a mission that we felt obliged to accept. In this endeavor, the assistance of many others who have cancer or have cared for loved ones, and have shared their stories with us, has helped us to tell ours.

We have also been helped enormously in this task by Jacqueline Wehmueller, executive editor at the Johns Hopkins University Press. Jackie recognized the value of what we wanted to do, in spite of our first attempt to describe it, and worked with us to shape this final product and to shepherd it through the Press's approval process. We are grateful to her. We also would like to thank all the other Hopkins Press staff members who have worked hard to bring this project to fruition. We especially thank Anne Whitmore, our manuscript editor, for her expertise and guidance in making our book so much more comprehensible, accurate, and readable than when she first received it.

Michael would like to express his gratitude to his wife, Elizabeth Bellamy. Beth has been the model of a caregiver—loving, supportive, watching over his welfare like a hawk—and without her he would surely not have made it this far. Michael also thanks his team at Johns Hopkins Hospital, led by Dr. Le, without whom, he has little doubt, he would not be here.

Dung would like to thank Michael for his vision and perseverance, without which this book would never have come to be. She would like to thank her husband, Henry Sun, whose concern for his patient brought Michael to her attention. She would like to express her appreciation to her mentors and colleagues, who serve as role models as they care for their patients in a compassionate manner and as they strive to advance the field of pancreatic cancer research.

Finally, Michael and Dung would like to thank all of the cancer patients and their families who serve as inspiration not only for this book but for continuing endeavors in research in hopes of benefiting future patients.

PANCREATIC CANCER

A Patient & His Doctor Balance Hope & Truth

1

The Gathering Clouds

B y all rights, I should not be here.

In December 2007, I was diagnosed with stage IV pancreatic cancer. The odds of someone with this cancer surviving for this long are very small indeed.

My oncologist, Dr. Dung Le, and my wife, Beth Bellamy, are my companions and guides on this journey. Our goal is to make it as long and as comfortable a trip as possible.

So far, we have succeeded.

Here is how we are going to tell our story. Dr. Le will alternate chapters with me. We will incorporate the experiences of many other people. We hope to make this a useful book for all who work with or are trying to come to grips with this disease. We also hope it will help people with other kinds of cancer, especially cancers with high mortality rates.

THE EARLY BACKGROUND

My wife and I met in 2002, married in 2003, and moved that same year from the suburbs of Washington, D.C., to Shepherdstown, West Virginia, a small college town about 70 miles from D.C. We were both in our sixties by then, but still healthy. People would sometimes say how young we looked, after they learned how old we really were. Perhaps they were being kind, but we enjoyed hearing this.

Still, I was 20 pounds overweight and had been taking medication for high cholesterol for several years. I also had been diagnosed with sleep apnea and had struggled, unsuccessfully, with using the facemask that had been prescribed.

The journey recounted in this book began with a number of signs. Most of them probably had nothing to do with cancer. They certainly meant I was growing older.

In 2005, I developed numbness in my big toe. There appeared to be, and there is still, no explanation for this. I also had several episodes of swelling of my ankles. I began to lose hearing in one ear. I was slightly anemic. A brain scan to see whether I might have a tumor that could be causing my loss of hearing showed instead that I was losing frontal lobe cells. An Internet search convinced me that I had Pick's Disease, a particularly severe form of dementia. My neurologist gently disabused me of that idea and told me to stop surfing the Internet.

My father had colon cancer, so my brother and I had had colonoscopies every few years since we turned 40. In the summer of 2007, I scheduled my first in almost five years. The result was a clean bill of health for the colon.

My big health news that summer of 2007, for which I will be forever grateful, was that during a routine exam a physician's assistant noticed that I had a heart murmur. I went forward with the obligatory ultrasound, in my local hospital. The diagnosis was an enlarged aortic root, and further assessment by a cardiologist was recommended.

My wife's childhood pediatrician, nearing 90 and by then a friend, had graduated from the Johns Hopkins School of Medicine. When we asked her where she would suggest I go for treatment, she said, "Why not go to Hopkins?" We liked this idea. Hopkins has a fine reputation and is only slightly farther away than the next best alternative. That was how we ended up in Baltimore, which is a 90-minute drive from home.

Having now talked with many people who are seriously ill or are caregivers, I've learned why more people do not go to a place like Hopkins. It might be too long a trip. It might be too expensive. However, another reason, based on these conversations, is that many people do not go to a major medical center because that is just not what they think to do when they are sick, even when seriously ill. If a doctor does not suggest going elsewhere for treatment, it is probably not going to happen. This is too bad, because in some cases there is real value in going a little farther from home.

Of course, many cancers can and should be treated close to home. I am not advocating that everyone immediately run to a teaching hospital. However, it is important to look at the alternatives.

In some cases, the person diagnosed, or the caregiver, does not accept their local doctor's opinion that there is nothing more to be done. Instead, they insist on going to another hospital. Looking elsewhere is not a panacea, it does not always lead to anything different, but sometimes it does help. In my case, it did.

Going to Hopkins meant meeting Dr. Henry Sun. The first time we saw Dr. Sun, he looked almost like a teenager to us. Beth and I felt so old. But what a good decision it was to go to Baltimore. Dr. Sun . . . Henry, as he insisted we call him . . . was calm, calming, and competent. He was also the first doctor I ever had who e-mailed me.

Henry ordered another ultrasound of my heart. I accepted this as a normal double-checking. He did not mistrust the earlier results but wanted to be careful. A second look can pick up things that might have been missed before. I welcomed the exam.

The second ultrasound confirmed the first. Henry said we should monitor the situation and see how, or if, things changed over the next several months and even years. Then we would know better whether it was necessary to do anything or we could afford to continue to wait. It seemed like a fairly ordinary and common happening.

We returned to Shepherdstown reassured. I learned all about the aortic root on the Internet, and then two months later went in for one more ultrasound. Nothing had changed, and we agreed to keep on watching it.

So there I was in the fall of 2007. It seemed to me, when I looked back on this time, that almost everything in my body had been falling apart. Certainly, I felt like almost every part of my body had been scanned. However, the part that really needed to be looked at hadn't been. This is sometimes what happens. No symptoms had pointed directly to the abdomen.

THE FIRST REAL SIGNS

In November 2007, I began to experience a persistent, aching feeling in my upper abdomen. I had lost 7 or 8 pounds since the summer, but I had been trying to lose weight, so that seemed good. I thought I was doing well. I learned later that this happens more often than one might think; people think they are doing well to lose weight, only to find that they are ill. Many people reported this to me when they recounted their own stories.

The pain was a dull ache, not sharp or acute, more like a presence that never went away. It would get better at night but it always returned. We went to see our new family doctor, Dr. Kinland, someone we have grown to respect and value, who prescribed something, but who also added, thank goodness, that if I did not feel better in a week I should get an abdominal scan. He gave me the order for it so that I would not have to return. He got the ball rolling.

The pain did not go away.

I had the scan in Frederick, Maryland. Everything was easy. The machine was just as I had always seen on TV. A cylinder that whirred as you passed through the donut ring. It took no time at all.

We were apprehensive but did not speculate. Beth might have had her suspicions; I had no idea. The results came back on my birthday, November 28th. They were not the present I was looking for. There were many spots in the pancreas and liver.

I did not know what to think. The best way to put it is that I was numb. I knew vaguely that pancreatic cancer was almost always fatal, usually quickly, and that anything down in that area was dangerous. Something in the liver was not much better. I did not know much more. My ignorance of what was happening became a recurring theme.

THE BIOPSY

Slightly dazed, I depended on others to tell me what the next step should be. My reaction was normal. This is exactly what happens to most people. The world is being turned upside down. Mine certainly was.

The urgent need at this point was to have a biopsy of the liver. Cancer does not typically begin in the liver. Having the liver biopsied is a way to document that cancer has spread to the liver and to pinpoint the source.

I was unable to have a biopsy immediately. We tried to book one at the hospital where I had had the scan, but they were full up, scheduled in advance for three weeks. This was the first time I ran up against a bottleneck in my health care.

Beth was fierce in insisting that we do something without delay. She has said since that she immediately went into a fighting mode. The moment we were told the scan results, she became the caregiver, ever vigilant. She brooked no delays. When this delay threatened, she went right back to Dr. Kinland. He found a hospital near Washington, they said to come, and we went down there the next day. However, I was unable to have the biopsy. The staff prepared me for the procedure, but because I had been taking a low dose of aspirin, my blood would not coagulate quickly enough for the biopsy needle to be safely inserted into my liver.

When we got home that evening, there was an e-mail waiting from Dr. Sun. At Beth's suggestion, I had e-mailed him that morning, saying that I had what appeared to be cancer in my liver and my pancreas, that I thought this probably would mean something for my heart treatment, and that we were having a problem scheduling the biopsy. I had asked him if he had suggestions as to what to do. He immediately wrote back to say that I should come to Hopkins for the biopsy. Also, he said, his wife, Dr. Le, was an oncologist, specializing in the pancreas.

Our spirits went up a bit. Something would be done. Because of my unrelated heart condition and because we had reached out as widely as possible, we had started down the road we now travel. Reflecting on this later, Beth observed that, while we knew in general how to go about in the medical world, we did not know, in the case of very serious illness, how in practical terms to get the treatment I needed. And even though I was well insured, so money was not a problem, we did not know exactly what to do.

Dr. Le had asked to see my scan before scheduling the biopsy. We called the hospital where it had been done, and they said they could give us a CD of it. Rather than wait until the hospital sent it on to Dr. Le (we were worried this might take extra time and that the CD might get lost), we decided to go to Frederick, pick it up ourselves, and take it to Baltimore directly. We did not want any more delays.

We drove the next day from home to the hospital that had done the abdominal scan, about 45 minutes away, picked up the CD, and continued on to Baltimore, another 45-minute drive. We did not talk much. We were focused on doing what we had to do. It felt like heading into a school examination unprepared. Beth recalls that Henry had given us his cell phone number, and as we neared Hopkins she called him. He came down and we met outside one of the buildings at the hospital. It was cold outside and he was not dressed warmly. He took the CD. We did not exchange many words. There just wasn't much to say. He did tell Beth to stay off the Internet. We drove home, satisfied that things were happening.

Within a day, I received a call from Hopkins telling me the biopsy was scheduled for the following week.

We came into Baltimore the day before the biopsy, stayed overnight in a hotel, and arrived early the next morning at the hospital. We headed into the bowels of the hospital's main building.

Everything was dreamlike. Everything and everyone moved right along, but it seemed like they were floating around me. I was there, but not there, not really present. I was lucky that Beth was with me. At least one of us is aware of everything that's going on, I thought.

I remember being prepared for the procedure. The Hopkins clinicians would do it using an ultrasound in real-time to guide the needle into the liver and to draw out the cells to be tested. This was a different procedure from the one that had been planned at the first hospital. There, they had intended using scanning to guide the needle insertion.

Once I was called in from the waiting area, everything went quickly. The team doing the biopsy gradually materialized out of nowhere, coming in one at a time, a few minutes apart, each getting busy immediately. They were well practiced. The procedure was explained to me. I was given a local anesthetic, Beth was invited in to watch, and the show got under way.

Everything depended on getting a sufficiently large sample and the right sample to be able to do the test. A specialist, a pathologist, was called in to confirm that the sample that had been withdrawn was adequate. He arrived immediately after being called. The team members were all sympathetic and knew exactly what they were doing. No second tries were needed. Everything was good.

That is, everything was good . . . except the results. These were, unfortunately, conclusive. I had cancer of the pancreas, and it was stage IV.

This was the worst news possible. It was as bad as bad could be. Not only was it stage IV, but the blood marker that signaled pancreatic cancer activity, something called CA19-9, was off the charts, at around 5000. A week earlier it had been half that. A normal reading is between 0 and 36. A week before I had not heard of this blood test, but I was learning quickly.

I remember feeling as if I was on a fast moving train, and all I could think was that I did not like where it was going. Being on a train or seeing a train became a familiar description as I listened to other patients' stories. It made sense in many ways. You do not have any control of the train when you are a passenger. It moves methodically forward. There is usually no way to get off. It sometimes stops and starts for no apparent reason.

After the biopsy was finished, we had been told that we would have the results in about a week, but a call came the very next day saying that I should come in as soon as possible. We were both apprehensive, but we were glad that things were moving along.

THE DIAGNOSIS

We met Dr. Le on the Monday after the biopsy. I do not remember very much from that first meeting. I do remember that Dr. Le was even younger looking than her husband. They *both* looked like teenagers.

Beth had taken a notebook along, luckily, and she took notes of what was said. Dr. Le told us about the alternative treatments that were available for pancreatic cancer, none of which sounded promising. Surgery was out of the question, as was radiation, because the cancer had already spread to the liver, where there were multiple tumors. Beth, who had looked at the sonogram when the biopsy was performed, has since told me that the liver looked like a piece of raisin bread.

Dr. Le—her first name is Dung (pronounced young)—was direct and serious. But she was also calm and reassuring in a certain way. She seemed to be someone we could trust, as well as someone who knew what she was talking about. Of course, we wanted to trust her.

She told us that stage IV cancer of the pancreas was not curable. The best that might be hoped for with treatment was to slow it down.

In the space of a minute, the way I thought about my life turned upside down. Just the week before, Beth and I had been talking about trips we might make in the future to visit grandchildren living in Africa and New Zealand, and other places we had always wanted to visit. I had been thinking about taking on more work as a consultant.

I thought all that had changed forever.

2

What Is Pancreatic Cancer and What Are Its Symptoms?

When I first heard that my husband, Henry, had a cardiology patient with abdominal pain, a pancreatic mass, and multiple liver lesions, numbers one, two, and three on my list of possible diagnoses were pancreatic adenocarcinoma. However, before giving someone such a diagnosis we must confirm it with a biopsy, because on rare occasions the diagnosis could be a category of pancreatic cancers called neuroendocrine cancer, or it could be a cancer metastasized from another organ, or sometimes it is even a non-cancer diagnosis. Neuroendocrine tumors deserve special mention, because they arise from a different cell type and carry a better prognosis than pancreatic adenocarcinomas. Michael's liver biopsy confirmed a diagnosis of metastatic pancreatic adenocarcinoma.

There were an estimated 43,140 new cases of pancreatic cancer diagnosed in the United States in 2010.[1] Unfortunately, the number of deaths due to pancreatic cancer nearly equals the number of new cases of the disease diagnosed each year. Pancreatic cancer is the fourth leading cause of cancer-related death in the United States. One of the reasons for this high mortality rate is that in 80 percent of patients the disease is diagnosed at an advanced stage. Most cancers are curable only if they are localized and can be surgically removed. Most patients with pancreatic cancer are diagnosed with advanced disease, in which cancer cells have migrated outside of the pancreas and surrounding lymph nodes and into other organs, such as the liver. This is what we refer to as *metastatic disease*. Even when the disease is only "locally advanced," confined to the region of the pancreas and the surrounding lymph nodes, surgery is not possible, because of involvement of the major abdominal blood vessels in the area of the pancreas.

The stage of a cancer describes the extent of advancement of the cancer. For pancreas cancer, stages IA through IIA include cancers that do not involve the lymph nodes. Stage IIB denotes lymph node involvement. At stages IA through IIB the disease is surgically operable; the status of the lymph nodes is not known until after the surgery. Stage III indicates a pancreatic tumor that involves the celiac axis or the superior mesenteric artery. These are major abdominal blood vessels, and their involvement usually means that the primary tumor is inoperable. Finally, metastatic disease, which has spread to other organs, is classified as stage IV.

The stage of disease at diagnosis has implications for the patient's prognosis and survival. Patients whose tumors have been surgically removed have a median survival of 17-24 months and a 5-year survival of approximately 20 percent. Patients with locally advanced disease have a median survival of 8-12 months. And patients with metastatic disease have a median survival of 4-6 months.

SIGNS AND SYMPTOMS

The story of Michael's diagnosis is not unusual for a patient with pancreatic cancer. Like a majority of patients, he was diagnosed with advanced disease. One of the reasons patients don't see their physicians until late in the course of the disease is that symptoms often do not appear until late in the course of the disease. Also, the symptoms are often rather vague, such as abdominal bloating, vague upper abdominal or back pain, weight loss, indigestion, and diarrhea, and can result from many different conditions. Most patients with these symptoms do not have pancreatic cancer. They are frequently diagnosed with more common disorders, such as gallstone disease or gastroesophageal reflux disease (heartburn). In addition, because the pancreas sits in front of the spine, the pain can be mistaken for muscle or arthritis pain. Often, further evaluation is pursued only after persistent weight loss and pain, and in many cases, only after the patient develops an elevated level of the bile pigment bilirubin, causing jaundice and a visible yellowing of the skin.

The jaundice and often-late onset of vague symptoms may be better understood in the context of the location of the pancreas (see Figure 2.1). The pancreas sits in the back of the upper abdomen, behind the stomach, in an area called the *retroperitoneum*. Depending on where the tumor starts, and especially if it is in the tail of the pancreas, it may not press on any adjacent structures and cause symptoms until it is relatively large or has already metastasized. In addition, a growth in the pancreas may not cause symptoms linked with the pancreas, such as pancreatitis (inflammation of the pancreas) or diabetes (a result of destruction of insulin producing cells) to raise a physician's suspicion of any pancreas-related disorder. However, a diagnosis of diabetes does often precede the diagnosis of pancreatic cancer.

Figure 2.1 shows why patients tend to develop jaundice when their tumors are located in the head of the pancreas. The common bile duct meets the pancreatic duct at the ampulla of vater and drains into the small bowel near the head of the pancreas. If a tumor is pressing on the exit path for the bile, it backs up, and the bilirubin in the blood and urine becomes elevated, resulting in itching, light-colored stools, yellow discoloration of the skin and eyes, and darkening of the urine.

Another difficulty in the diagnosis of pancreatic cancer at earlier stages is that often the primary tumor is of small or moderate size but contains cells with a high propensity to metastasize. A patient may have metastatic disease despite having only a small primary tumor in the pancreas. This is one reason that at least 70 to 80 percent of patients who undergo a surgical resection, or removal, of the tumor still have a recurrence of the cancer. Although everyone hopes that the surgeon "got it all," there are often metastatic cells that have migrated to other organs but are not detectable even by our modern imaging tests. However, pancreatic cancer is not uniformly fatal. The flipside of this negative statistic is that 20 percent of patients who undergo removal of their cancers are long-term survivors.

Michael had been having epigastric pain, which is pain in the upper abdomen, for about one month and had been prescribed a medication to suppress the acid in his stomach, to treat possible heartburn or inflammation of the stomach. After his symptoms did not improve, a CT scan was obtained (see Figure 2.2), and it showed multiple liver masses and a lesion in the tail of the pancreas. His CA19-9, which is a tumor marker measured in the blood, was elevated to greater than 5000 units per milliliter. Not all pancreatic cancers cause an elevation in CA19-9. Elevated levels of the marker do not always indicate the presence of cancer, but the elevation in the CA19-9 was more evidence that Michael likely had a pancreatic adenocarcinoma. In addition, pancreatic tail cancers often are diagnosed later, because they are less likely to cause symptoms than head of the pancreas cancers, since they do not push on anything, such as the bile duct.

Michael had lost weight over the preceding months, which he attributed to successful dieting, an account we often hear from pancreatic cancer patients. He had smoked tobacco in the past, which is a risk factor for pancreatic cancer, and he is of Ashkenazi Jewish descent. There is an increased risk of pancreatic cancer in Ashkenazi Jews, which may be due to a variety of factors, such as smoking, diet, and/or inherited mutations such as mutations in the BRCA genes.

The results of the biopsy of the lesion on Michael's liver were consistent with a pancreatobiliary primary cancer. This means that

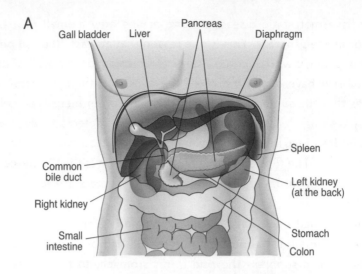

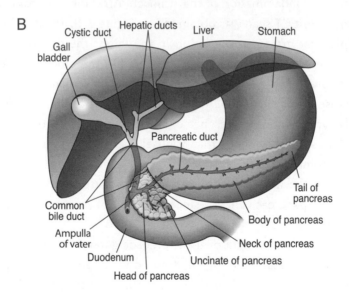

Figure 2.1 (*A*) Anatomy of the pancreas in the context of the abdomen. (*B*) Relationship of the pancreas to the duodenum, stomach, bile ducts, and liver.

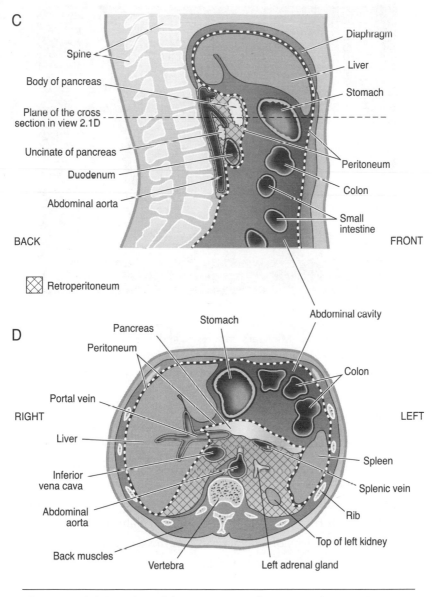

Figure 2.1 (*C*) Location of the pancreas in the retroperitoneum in vertical cross section. (*D*) Location of the pancreas in the retroperitoneum in horizontal cross section viewed from below.

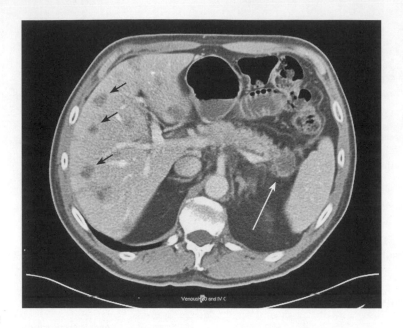

Figure 2.2 CT scan of Michael's pancreatic and liver tumors at the time of diagnosis. The black arrows point to some of the tumors that spread to his liver; the white arrow points to the primary pancreatic tumor.

the cancer started in either the pancreas or the bile ducts. Given the pancreatic mass, liver lesions, and elevated CA19-9, his clinical diagnosis was consistent with pancreatic adenocarcinoma. Some risk factors and symptoms that he did not have were obesity, new onset diabetes, steatorrhea (floating stools due to malabsorption), history of pancreatitis, history of unexplained superficial or deep blood clots, ascites (abdominal fluid), or jaundice.

DIAGNOSIS AND PLANNING

The process of discussing a new diagnosis of metastatic pancreatic cancer with a patient and his family is never easy. Their lives have essentially been turned upside down and their long-term goals suddenly become unachievable. Physicians are never sure how much

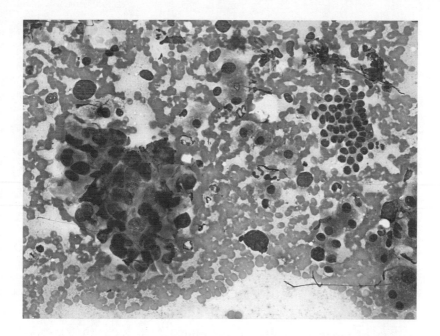

Figure 2.3 Biopsy of one of Michael's liver tumors. A dark clump of abnormally large and irregular cancer cells is visible at left amid normal liver cells. A cluster of benign, or non-cancerous, tumor cells, center right, shows size comparison.

information the patient and his family are really taking in. It is difficult to balance what a patient needs to hear and what a patient wants or is able to hear. Statistics must be quoted cautiously, so as not to overwhelm a patient who is not ready to hear the numbers. However, it is sometimes difficult to discuss the issue of prognosis with a patient and family if it was not disclosed during the initial consultation. I do feel that it is my obligation to the patient and the family to discuss prognosis, if they are ready, from the start, so that they are aware of realities, feel informed, and can plan their affairs accordingly. This is certainly a delicate process; it is not uncommon for patients to tell me that they had not returned to a physician's office because they were told that they had two months to live and to "get their affairs in order." While it is a cliché, I do use the phrase "plan for the worst and hope for the best."

As I do with other patients with metastatic pancreatic cancer, I told Michael and Beth that the median survival time for patients with metastatic disease is six months and that I did not have a crystal ball to predict exactly how long he would live. *Median* means that half the patients do worse and half the patients do better. For someone with Michael's diagnosis, after one year only 20 percent of patients would be alive. Our goal was *palliative*, not curative, treatment, meaning that we wanted to extend his life with the best quality of life possible but that we would not be able to eradicate the disease. We also discussed why surgical resection—removal—of the cancer was not an option. The cancer had already spread from the pancreas; in addition to his pancreatic masses, he had multiple liver lesions, which the biopsy had proven to be cancer. In fact, because of the biology of pancreatic cancer, even if he had had only a few lesions in his liver, it was likely that there were other metastatic lesions that we could not see by our imaging techniques.

As you can imagine, hearing this news for the first time, or even the tenth time, is difficult for any person. As part of their initial consultation, patients expect to learn not just about prognosis but also about treatment options. Metastatic pancreatic cancer is a systemic disease, meaning that the process is not localized to one area of the body. Treatment must also be systemic, targeting multiple areas of the body. In fact, a majority of patients whose pancreatic tumors are surgically removed have a recurrence of their cancer. They may have a local recurrence or one in another organ due to microscopic metastatic deposits that were present at the time of surgery but not visible.

The most common systemic treatment for cancer is chemotherapy. Each chemotherapy drug works by a slightly different mechanism, but in general, chemotherapeutic drugs interfere with DNA or cell division and repair. While a majority of chemotherapies act on all dividing cells, the rapidly dividing cells of cancer are the most affected.

Metastatic disease is typically treated with chemotherapy alone (the topic of chemotherapy options is discussed further in Chapter 4). An appendix is also provided at the back of this book for those who would like more detailed information on the origin of cancer cells and a summary of therapeutic approaches to the various stages of pancreatic cancer other than metastatic disease. This background may be useful, because at initial consultations most patients and their families have a series of questions about why or how the patient developed the cancer and why, unfortunately, it is usually not operable. In truth, it is often the family members who ask the initial questions, as many patients are somewhat numb for a while after hearing their diagnosis.

I explained to Michael and Beth before we embarked on his therapy that the goals of the chemotherapy would be to improve or maintain his quality of life and to prolong survival and that we would work together to find a balance between these goals.

3

The Fight Begins

CHOOSING A TREATMENT AND
A PLACE TO BE TREATED

Choosing a Treatment

I n December 2007 Beth and I sat in Dr. Le's office after being told I had stage IV pancreatic cancer. I was scared to ask what came next.

Dr. Le was calm. We were in a small cubicle, equipped with a desk and computer, one of many in which bad news, and sometimes good, is delivered. I do not remember much more than that. Beth and I sat together on one side of the desk. Dung had to look back and forth to include both of us. She took a breath and began what must also have been a painful process for her. But she had done this before, many times.

She outlined four alternatives. The first was the traditional treatment for pancreatic cancer—gemcitabine (Gemzar is its brand name). The second was gemcitabine combined with a targeted agent, Tarceva. I was not sure what "targeted agent" meant, but it seemed like a good idea to try to target the tumors. The third was a more aggressive, more experimental, treatment, a "cocktail" of chemotherapy drugs called GTX (Gemzar, Taxotere, and Xeloda). I remember thinking, isn't there a motor oil like that?

At some point, we also talked about the possibility of my entering one of the studies of other therapies. The problem was that there were no studies that I could begin immediately. I might have had to wait as long as a month, and that was too long. Also, a study, to my way of thinking, meant experimenting, and this made me apprehensive. A study was not a realistic alternative for me.

The final option was to do nothing. Well, nothing more than try to manage the pain. The cancer was well-advanced. Chemotherapy was likely to be rough, and it might not prolong my life. I could opt for a relatively less painful, non-chemo-filled, final few months.

We did not really know what to think. We needed guidance. In truth, I wanted someone else to make the decision.

Beth tried another tack. She asked Dung what she would do if it were her husband. We understood she wanted us rather than her to make the decisions for my care, but we were trying to guess what she thought was best. We did not think about the differences between Henry and me. Later we recognized that, rightly or wrongly, we had wanted to believe that she was leaning toward GTX, the most aggressive of the treatments.

Beth and I looked at each other. We decided that both of us wanted the most aggressive treatment possible. We thought this to be GTX. I chose to begin GTX as soon as possible. I knew this was not a cure, but I wanted to do something.

As I think about this now, I realize that, in spite of all the advice about investigating and reading and talking to as many people as possible when you are diagnosed with cancer, doing so is sometimes very difficult. But shouldn't there always be a second opinion? I had always thought so, in the abstract. We could have obtained another opinion, but I thought we didn't have the time. The facts were clear. I was in a leading hospital. I wanted to act, not to wait. I felt that I had waited too long already.

I started GTX the next day.

All told, less than two weeks had passed between getting the results of my abdominal scan and starting my treatment. I had stage IV cancer, but I was being treated in one of the best medical places in the world.

Today, I can only wonder at how ignorant I was about what had happened and was going to happen. I knew very little about cancer and its treatment, and even less about the pancreas. I did not think much about it at the time. I was in shock. I relied on Beth and Dr. Le to guide me.

Recently, an acquaintance called me for advice about his upcoming visit to an oncologist. He had had cancer before and had been treated, but a subsequent scan revealed that his cancer had returned. We talked for about 45 minutes. He did not know very much, in spite of his earlier cancer and treatment. I asked Beth later if I had also been this short of information. Yes, came the answer.

In hindsight, however, there is no way I would have chosen a different treatment. And I believe that most people, even if it is clear that their odds of surviving for very long are slim, they are very much older, or they are convinced that their situation is hopeless, will want to try something, anything, at least for a while.

I think about others whose stories I now know who had been in this situation. Almost none of them began treatment as quickly as I did. It makes me believe that the key to good and possibly successful treatment that might prolong life is rapid diagnosis and taking immediate steps at a place where people know what they are doing. A place that is experienced in treating the particular kind of cancer with which you have been diagnosed.

However, this is not possible for everyone. I talked with a woman whose husband had delayed going to the doctor, thinking the ache in his stomach was something minor. He was a large man and his eventual examination did not reveal any tumors. The aches remained unexplained. By the time he went to a larger hospital, it was too late.

Another example concerns an acquaintance of mine who waited months in the face of serious symptoms before going to an oncologist. His primary physician did not diagnose possible cancer. The symptoms could have been caused by less serious conditions, and it is a mistake to rush to judgment. Still, nothing that was prescribed helped. He might also have been in some form of denial about the symptoms and not eager to find the real cause. Finally, he went to an oncologist. A test quickly revealed cancer. Surgery followed. We are hoping everything will work out for him. An earlier diagnosis might have made treatment easier.

Although it is often difficult to verify stories one reads on the Internet, some of them and others I have heard do confirm that acting quickly helps. I think this is common sense. I believe that acting quickly gave me a chance to prolong my life in those early months.

There have been many discussions about what hope means for people newly diagnosed with cancer. Inherent in my decision to try an aggressive treatment—undergirding it—was the hope that something might "work." What did "work" mean to me? Not a cure, even though I might have secretly hoped for this. It meant living reasonably well for as long as possible. I had no idea what chemotherapy might entail, but I doubt if anything could have deterred me pursuing it.

Not everyone chooses an aggressive treatment. Some have disease that is so advanced that the only treatment possible is pain management. They do not have a choice.

It never entered my mind that I would not fight. Looking back, my guess (I have to reconstruct this because I was in a fog at the time) is that even though stage IV pancreatic cancer usually portends a very short survival time, I wanted to live for as long as possible. I had things I wanted to do. Among them was that I had to put my affairs in order.

Jane Brody's *Guide to the Great Beyond*[1] tells the story of Anna Engquist, an 80-year-old who developed ovarian cancer and required major surgery. She also wanted to put her affairs in order. She was told that the surgery would be risky. In spite of her age and her general condition, she decided to go ahead. She spent the week before the surgery wrapping up things and saying goodbye to loved ones. She even left a note on the kitchen table before going to the hospital for the operation, describing the regular bills that needed to be paid and listing the repairs needed in the house. She knew she might not come back. It was important to her that people know what to do in her absence. Anna's story has a good ending. She survived the operation and the very difficult chemotherapy that followed.

Of course, there are people who do not pursue treatment because they would not be able to withstand the impact of chemotherapy, being already too weak. There are those who, believing that their time has come, decide to forgo chemotherapy. It is a deeply personal decision.

Dr. Sherwin Nuland writes movingly in *How We Die*[2] about his brother Harvey, who was dying from intestinal cancer that had metastasized. Dr. Nuland, a surgeon and professor, wrote that he had counseled many patients about end-of-life decisions and that he strongly favored being as honest as possible in telling patients their odds of survival with and without treatment, to the extent that these odds are known. During surgery, it was confirmed that the cancer had spread extensively. Dr. Nuland could not bring himself to tell his brother that there were no known drugs or procedures that could prevent his death within the next several months. Instead, he proposed an experimental approach. The result was a painful period of chemotherapy, followed by death. Although he had been fairly certain that this was going to happen, he could not bring himself to destroy the hope his brother had. Dr. Nuland came to believe that his brother would have been more comfortable had he chosen not to receive treatment. He probably would have lived roughly the same amount of time.

I was not old. I did not have unbearable symptoms. My desire was to do whatever might be possible to extend my life a little. My decisions were based on this desire. That we had never heard of GTX did not matter. There would be time to learn about it later.

We had been cautioned about Internet searches, many of which turn up incorrect and alarming opinions. I usually limited myself to reading university, government, or nonprofit sites. We looked up GTX as soon as we could. We found it had been used in a study on 35 patients at Columbia University, about five or six years earlier.

That was all that we could find online about it. GTX really was experimental. The implications became more real. Although not participating in a study, I was to be on the cutting edge of something that had not progressed beyond that one trial at Columbia.

The statistics were sobering. GTX seemed somewhat promising, from what I knew about survival rates. However, it was difficult to confirm this without knowing much more than I found on the Internet. One thing was crystal clear. After three years, very few of the participants were alive. This was sobering.

The final report on the study had been written earlier that year, 2007.[3] Although the numbers did suggest some advantage in taking GTX, it was clearly not a silver bullet. It did not cure. It was not suitable, as I understood it, for many people, especially those who were not relatively strong.

All this knowledge came gradually, after we had made our decision.

Choosing the Johns Hopkins Hospital and the Kimmel Cancer Center

When my diagnosis happened, we had been in the middle of remodeling our home. We felt we could not continue that project. We decided to move instead, to a cottage nearby that would be easier to manage. We canceled plans to go to North Carolina for Christmas and the celebration of Beth's mother's birthday. Beth canceled her December trip to Chicago, where she went quarterly for migraine headache treatments. She has had terrible migraines for many years. She put my health first.

Beginning chemotherapy was uppermost in our minds. We thought that if anything could be done, it would be done at Johns Hopkins. We gave little thought to alternative treatments or locations.

Hopkins has been rated the number one hospital in the United States for twenty straight years by *U.S. News and World Report*. One of the hospital's particular areas of expertise is pancreatic cancer. Does this mean that Hopkins is better than the Mayo Clinic, the Cleveland Clinic, MD Anderson, or any of another six or eight cancer centers? Perhaps not. It may be meaningless to make such a comparison. They are all top-notch. In any event, I have always been skeptical of these kinds of ratings by magazines. Hopkins is a world-class institution. Whether it was first or not, its proximity to our home in West Virginia made Hopkins the best choice for us.

However, for all its renown, Hopkins is a real life, fairly gritty, not in the least luxurious big-city hospital. Actually, it mirrors the city of Baltimore. When I lived in Washington, I liked to drive over to Baltimore for the day. It is more like a real city to me than Washington, with its overwhelmingly governmental character.

Nurses, doctors, orderlies, and patients bustle about. Sick people are wheeled around the corridors. This is not a health spa. In fact, it is the exact opposite. It is smack in the middle of some of the most depressed parts of Baltimore. Looking at Hopkins from other parts of the city, it rises above its surroundings, a mixture of the old and the new, the past and the future, gleaming in its massiveness. Physically, it invites confidence.

Inside, there is a feeling in the air that good things are happening. There are signs on the walls everywhere with the objectives of the hospital. Helping people is the primary objective. The attitude of every worker in the hospital we met reflected the healing philosophy.

We had noticed during my cardiology visits that there was a suite of offices dedicated to visitors from overseas. This was our first indication that Hopkins was different. Later, as I underwent chemo, we would occasionally see an interpreter accompanying a patient visiting from abroad. We would also see people at our hotel who had flown in for treatment from Florida, Alaska, and foreign countries.

When we arrived for the first chemo treatment, we went directly to the Kimmel Comprehensive Cancer Center, a new part of the hospital complex. In the Kimmel Center, there was far less bustling about. It was much quieter. There was less palpable optimism in the air. Or maybe that was only my perspective. It was a sobering beginning.

TREATMENT, REACTIONS, AND NEXT STEPS

The Treatment Process

The first thing I did when I went for treatments was check in. Everything is computerized. The computer will either confirm your appointments and print out a schedule, or ask you to see the admin office if there is a problem. Following check-in, my next stop was to have blood drawn at the phlebotomy lab, on the same floor but around the corner. We would usually need to wait a few minutes for that. The technician behind the desk, Walter, came to know my name and would greet me when I came into the lab waiting room. This surprised me at first. He must see literally scores of patients every day, I thought. It is a small but important expression of interest and care from the first level of staff whom a patient encounters in the hospital. The blood would be drawn, blood pressure taken, temperature and pulse measured. There was usually a lot of banter among the technicians. Even so, this is a serious place. The process never varied.

We would then go upstairs to the chemo waiting room. Every new area we entered required a scan of my hospital card. This allows the staff in each area to know that the patient is there and ready to be seen.

The results of the blood tests determine whether chemo will be given that day. Blood has to be analyzed to make sure that the body is strong enough to handle the chemo. If my white blood cell count dipped too low, I might not be given additional chemotherapy drugs until my blood counts rose to acceptable levels. We learned a new vocabulary, with words such as creatinine, bilirubin, neutrophils, and platelets. When my creatinine went up, we began to worry. We learned to watch these numbers.

All of this keeps most people in the waiting room a little bit on edge until they receive the signal that chemo can proceed. Once the nurse gives the green light, the pharmacy lab folks mix the correct amounts of each drug for that day. The whole process from the taking of blood to the analysis to the preparation of the chemos usually takes a couple of hours.

The first time we went for my treatment, the time in the waiting room upstairs seemed interminable. The room lived up to its name. Everyone just waited. It was a comfortable room, but far from luxurious. The furniture was old; there were no frills. There was a TV but, thank goodness, no sound. In the beginning there were very soothing scenes of nature on the television. Unfortunately, about six months into my treatments someone found the remote control and changed the setting to a news channel and turned on the sound. After that, we had to endure that most common of all waiting room amenities, the droning background TV.

The condition of my fellow patients varied. Some were obviously ill, some fairly healthy looking. Some were wearing gauze surgical masks. Most were not.

We became friends with a few of the couples we saw every week. People supported each other, shared whatever good news there might be, and commiserated with one another over setbacks. People in such waiting rooms understand that everyone there is confronting life and death issues. Beth, more often than I, has reached out to meet others and has felt support from our waiting room friends; but I have talked to a couple of patients who were beginning GTX, telling them my experience, and this seems to provide some comfort to them.

Some patients have learned that their initial treatments were not as successful as hoped, and they come to chemotherapy realizing that their prognosis is not as good.

Over the course of treatment visits, some patients did not come back. This was a reminder of what was going on. We came to know who was being treated for pancreatic cancer and would notice when he or she did not come back. We would know that probably the treatment was not working.

A volunteer comes at 10 on Fridays and asks everyone if they want something to drink, or a snack. It is a nice touch.

On the day of the first treatment, the wait for the therapy itself seemed long. Finally I was called. Beth and I went together into what we came to learn is called a chemotherapy pod. Perhaps ten to twelve patients receive treatment at the same time in a pod. There are four pods surrounding the waiting room. This means that there are up to nearly fifty people, connected under the umbrella of a diagnosis of cancer, being treated at any one time.

The pod is an endlessly interesting place. At each of the chairs or beds a scene is played out. Sometimes the person receiving chemo is alone, but more often there is a companion. The faces tell stories of care and hope. There are old couples who have probably had a lifetime together. There are younger couples, sometimes with children. There are whites and blacks, gay couples, sisters and brothers, and just plain friends. The patients generally rest when receiving chemotherapy. Those who come with the patients may bring computers, knitting, or books. Sometimes, both the patient and his or her companion just rest. The companions lend their support and show their love simply by being there.

The pod is a place that renders everyone equal. There are the poor and the well-to-do, sitting side by side. It makes no difference. We are all sick, all going through the same process, all equal.

That first morning, we met two people who would become integral and intense parts of our lives. Paula Lavelle is the oncology nurse who works with many of Dr. Le's patients, and Linda Taylor is the pod's clinical associate, in charge of inserting the IVs and doing a dozen other things that make the place run smoothly. These two people became part of our family as we became part of the Hopkins family. They, like Dr. Le, are the faces of the institution. They inspire confidence. They clearly know what they are doing. They are sympathetic and quietly cheerful.

Also in the pod are four other wonderful oncology nurses, who work as a team with Paula and Linda: Suzanne Hoffert, Margaret Gardner, Ella Mae Shupe, and Jane Diaz. The place is active, efficiently run, and usually cheerful. Thank goodness for this team and this place is all I can say now.

I do not recall ever having had an IV before my chemotherapy. I did break my elbow when I was 15, and I might have had one then, but I cannot remember; that was almost fifty years ago. I was on edge before the first treatment began.

I settled into a reclining chair next to the nurses' station. I think they put people in that particular chair the first time they have chemo in order to watch for problems and reactions. In later visits, I would go to a window alcove perch where I could look out the window at the traffic below, and I would feel a sense of calm. That first December day, it was raining and gray outside. Linda wheeled up her materials and the ever-present machine that would control the infusion. She bent over my arm and gently felt here and there, trying to make sure to find the right vein. She invariably does. She inserted the intravenous needle. Along with the two bottles of liquid Taxotere and Gemzar (Xeloda is taken as a pill, by mouth), there are bags of hydrating liquid and some sort of steroid. I never did completely understand how the steroid works, only that it is supposed to, and does, make everything happen a little better. At that time, I did not understand how chemotherapy works. In general, I understood that the drugs attack fast-growing cells, but that was about all I knew.

Everything is efficient, everyone is friendly. Although it feels like the treatments take a long time, the span of time is actually reasonable. In at 8 o'clock for the blood draw, in the waiting room by 9, in the pod by 11, and finished by early afternoon.

Beth usually takes a chair next to me, and sometimes gets out something to read. She usually brings a laptop. She may get me coffee, juice, or something from the cafeteria. Sometimes she talks with other patients and the nurses, when we have a question regarding my care. She gets together the printouts that detail the results of all my blood tests, and we pore over these, trying to discern some sort of trend. I doze quite a bit of the time I am receiving the drugs.

The schedule for chemotherapy is rigid. I try to stick to it. I believe this is important. My regimen requires two weeks on chemo and one week off. During the two weeks on, I take Xeloda twice a day and get IV chemo each Friday. For the IV treatments, we drive to Baltimore and stay over for one or two nights. Every third week, we get to stay at home.

The Effects of Chemo

During my first year after diagnosis, I went through 21 cycles of chemotherapy—that's 42 weeks on and 21 weeks off. I missed only three IV sessions; we came to Hopkins, but my white blood cell counts were too low for me to safely withstand the chemo assault.

Being able to keep up the schedule has been important, I feel. We saw that some of my fellow patients could not withstand the rigorous schedule. Chemotherapy targets all cells that are fast growing. It also destroys not only cancer cells but your bone marrow, over time. This leads to a reduction in red and white blood cells and so a decrease in strength and in the effectiveness of the immune system. Some people's systems cannot recover quickly enough from one week's chemotherapy to be able to have the next week's round.

Then there are those rare individuals who hold up under treatment for years. One person I talked with has metastatic breast cancer and had been treated non-stop for more than six years—two weeks on, two weeks off now, although the regimen has changed over time. I recently read on the CancerCompass Web site[4] about someone who has pancreatic cancer and has been on GTX for almost six straight years. Surviving for that long and being on chemo without a rest seems amazing to me.

The opposite sometimes happens, and it is because chemotherapy can be rough. A friend of ours in Shepherdstown, who had breast cancer almost ten years ago, told us that after her surgery and radiation she could not continue with the chemotherapy because it was just too brutal. At that time there were not as many drugs to mitigate bad reactions as now. She made the difficult decision to stop treatment. She survived. Subsequently, when she developed a different kind of cancer, she was able, with the help of new drugs, to control the nausea and to successfully complete her chemotherapy for the new cancer.[5]

If side effects, such as nausea, do not prevent treatment, the assault of the chemo on the bone marrow may, eventually. Our bone marrow produces red blood cells, white blood cells, and platelets. White cells fight infection, and platelets allow blood to clot. Red cells carry oxygen throughout the body. Each function is crucial.

My white blood cell count dropped, as did my red blood cell count. On two separate occasions, I had to have blood transfusions. The worst part for me was the sinking feeling that chemo had to be postponed. I believed that keeping to my schedule was one of the keys to surviving longer and feeling better. Anything that prevented me from doing this meant, to me, that I might be losing ground that I would never be able to recover.

There is not an easy remedy when white cell counts sink too low. Below a certain level, a person can no longer take the chemo. Luckily, this happened to me only three times.

Beth and I began to read about research that holds the promise of a more targeted approach to attacking cancer cells. Some day it might be possible to look at each individual's cancer and devise a treatment specifically for that particular case. This is an enormously complicated undertaking, but it holds the key to better results.

Chemotherapy today is more like a sledgehammer approach.

My side effects came immediately. They included overwhelming fatigue, a dry mouth as well as sores in my mouth, and the loss of all my hair. Actually, losing my hair did not bother me. I thought I looked better! Then there were the dry, cracked feet that needed to be kept constantly smothered in various creams.

I also had constipation. I much preferred that to the opposite, diarrhea. I felt just plain awful. I lost my appetite. Everything tasted funny.

However, I was lucky. Although I was nauseated at times, I never threw up. When I did feel queasy, I took Zofran. This amazing little pill is effective for me, although it might not do the trick for everyone.

I had lost almost 10 pounds before being diagnosed. I had been watching my weight, so thought I was doing great, until the pain began in November. I lost another 20 pounds before stabilizing at around 155 pounds. That meant I lost nearly 30 pounds in all.

The change in my taste buds came almost immediately. I might like something for a week or two, and then not like it. At different times, I might crave something like orange juice. Then, suddenly, my taste for it would disappear. Sometimes food tasted metallic. Mostly it did not have much taste.

Mouth sores proved to be a serious side effect. Sometimes it was almost impossible to swallow anything. Luckily, my disinterest in food did not extend to a childhood favorite of mine, Spaghettios. I still liked the taste and they slid down my throat with almost no effort. I ate so much of the product that some friends from down the road, Tony and Donna, came by with a gift of cans of Spaghettios, but the alphabet-shaped kind. They joked that I needed a change of diet.

Beth worked hard to interest me in different foods. She strongly believes in keeping my weight up, even if the food is not particularly healthful. Looking back, I think this is the right approach. I am not counseling anyone to abandon healthy eating habits. I am saying that we thought it more important to keep my weight up than to worry about whether a diet with considerable fat in it would cause my cholesterol to increase. At that point, we were more focused on my cancer than on my heart.

For my initial abdominal pain, Dr. Le prescribed 10 mg of Oxy-Contin (oxycodone), twice a day, and this was immediately effective. As the chemotherapy began to work, I believe the tumors became smaller and ceased pressing against whatever had then caused the pain. I suspected that I needed the drug less.

After two years on OxyContin, I decided it was time to wean my-self off it. This decision came from my beginning to have confidence that I would be alive for a while longer. Previously I had reasoned that it made no sense to stop taking the pain killer if the tumors were going to resume their growth. I began by not taking the morn-ing dose. The only time I really felt bad was after I stopped taking the evening dose; I had trouble trying to get to sleep without the pill. For several nights, I took Tylenol, and then I decided to go cold turkey. That sounds funny to say. My attempt to stop this powerful pain killer was only marginally like someone with a real addiction trying to get off a drug. Several more days and I was off OxyContin for the first time in two years. I have not experienced any pain since.

Many patients are not able to tolerate having the IV needle in-serted repeatedly for their chemo infusions. After a certain number of insertions, the veins may become scarred and close off. These patients require a "port," a small device that is surgically placed, usu-ally in the upper chest area. It provides a passageway for the direct infusion of the chemotherapy drug into the patient's body. This is a minor procedure, but the thought of it gives me the shivers, per-haps because, in my mind, I associate a port with a decline in my ability to receive chemotherapy, and also, perhaps paradoxically, with long-term, perhaps forever, treatment. I much prefer the nee-dle, and luckily my veins have thus far withstood the repeated sticks.

During those first two months of chemo I was reeling, physically and emotionally. Although I never threw up, I was almost always woozy and weak. I lost almost all stamina. Bending down to pick up my shoes or socks in an effort to be useful around the house would exhaust me.

Although I did not feel good immediately after chemo, I also did not feel horrible. I would feel bloated and uncomfortable for several days and generally lethargic. It was usually on the third or fourth day after chemo that the worst symptoms appeared. These included nausea, sometimes a slight fever, and generally a feeling of debilitation. These symptoms lasted undiminished for about a day and then gradually wore off.

Beth's care was critical to my treatment. She worried over me night and day. Sometimes, it seemed she slept with one eye open, watching me. She made charts of exactly when I had to take my pills, and we had to check off each dose as it was taken. She insisted to the hotel that we be given extra-quiet rooms. She made sure in the cold winter that we had blankets in the car for our trips to Baltimore. She hovered, protecting me.

When I began chemotherapy, I took oral steroids the day before, the day of, and the day after having chemo. Gradually, over the next few months, the dosage of oral steroids was reduced, but I continued to receive steroids by infusion with the chemotherapy. In June 2008, six months after starting chemo, Dr. Le decided to stop all oral steroids. Almost immediately, two days after having chemo, I woke up with a temperature nearing 100 degrees. It continued to climb throughout the day.

My marching orders were clear in such a situation. Because of the danger that the fever might be caused by an infection, and because my immune system was depressed from the chemo, I was to go to a hospital emergency room if my temperature went past the 100.4 mark. We rushed to the ER, but the doctors there could find nothing alarming. After a number of hours, and two Tylenol pills, I was sent home.

About three weeks later the same thing happened, with the same results. Dr. Le suggested it might be the cessation of the oral steroids, which had been mitigating some effects of the chemotherapy. Instead of restarting the oral steroids, which can have long-term undesirable effects, I began taking a very low dosage of Tylenol on the day of and the day after having chemotherapy, and I have not been to the ER since for an elevated temperature.

Realities of Treatment

The subject of the effects of chemotherapy needs to be put in perspective. Complications are part of the reality of cancer treatment, whether it is surgical, radiological, or chemical. Although the direct effects and side effects of chemotherapy are usually serious, people with pancreatic cancer who are treated with surgery, most often an operation called the Whipple, also face issues.

A person we know was able to have the Whipple operation, but complications from the surgery soon appeared. The stomach, small intestine, and pancreas had been reconfigured, so resuming even a relatively restricted diet was difficult. In addition, there were problems with the incision, which did not heal properly. A great number of Whipples are performed at Johns Hopkins Hospital every year, but even so, complications develop. For me, the lesson is that no matter which treatment a person has, there are going to be issues.

Much later, the reality of the statistics, no matter what the treatment was, sank in for me. About 80 percent of people diagnosed with pancreatic cancer are diagnosed with advanced cancer or for some other reason are unable to have surgery. For those in the remaining 20 percent who do have surgery, in 80 percent the cancer recurs.

Even so, being able to have surgery has better outcomes (a longer life expectancy), on average, than having chemotherapy only.

However, I was not a candidate for surgery because of the metastasis of cancer cells to the liver. I understood that had I been able to have the Whipple operation, it would have given me a greater chance of living longer. I did not fully appreciate this until I did further research later. On the Web site of the Pancreatic Cancer Action Network,[6] sometimes known as PanCAN, an organization that does much to promote awareness of pancreatic cancer, the vast majority of successful survival stories are from people who were able to have the Whipple surgery. There are very few success stories for people whose cancer has metastasized.

Family History and Risk Factors

One of the first pieces of mail I received from Johns Hopkins after my treatment had begun was a request that I participate in a survey and program[7] to trace my family's history of illnesses. I agreed to do this. I thought it might be of medical interest and potentially helpful to others in my family, longer term. By this time, I had read that Ashkenazi Jews, those who come from Eastern Europe, are more likely to develop pancreatic cancer. I have never been religious, but I am certainly an Ashkenazi Jew. I have one biological son, and three biological grandchildren, as well as a brother, sister, and many cousins. I solicited as much information as I could from my sister, brother, and uncle.

There had not been any pancreatic cancer in my immediate family that anyone knew of. However, both of my parents had had other types of cancer. My mother died with chronic leukemia. My father had been successfully treated for colon cancer. I had never thought about this before. When I did, it made sense that eventually I might also be diagnosed with some form of cancer. I had smoked when I was a teenager. Not heavily, and I had stopped in my late twenties, but there it was, I had smoked. Overall, I had not led an unhealthy life, but I guess I could have tried harder to reduce my risks for cancer.

I worried about my biological son and my grandchildren. I told him about all the things that might make a difference. Not smoking was the most important. Being aware that unexplained symptoms, like those I had noticed in the year before my diagnosis, might be a clue. Letting the doctor know the family history. Much later, I decided to undergo genetic testing for the most common type of mutant genes, BRCA 1 and 2. The results were negative.

I wonder about the role that stress plays in bringing on illness. I had been under a lot of stress in the fifteen years prior to my diagnosis. I had been through a divorce, counseling for a number of years, and a longish relationship that ended stressfully. I had remarried in 2003, but the second marriage had also had its difficulties.

The role of stress is difficult to gauge. Some studies show that people who have been through a divorce tend to have more medical problems, even if they remarry. I have read that there is no clear evidence that stress can lead directly to cancer. This makes sense to me, intuitively. After all, many people who live under tremendous strain do not develop cancer. Still, I wonder.

However, all I could do as I embarked on cancer therapy was deal with the present. None of this other stuff really mattered in the short term. I began to think about all I had to do in what might be a short period. My greatest concern was to put my affairs in order.

Having immediate tasks to do turned out to be helpful for me. I would come to see that having long-term goals was also therapeutic.

Although there is now much information—and misinformation— available to lay people about cancer, I had not obsessed about knowing as much as doctors about pancreatic cancer. Of course, I read a lot, but I avoided the blogs and the Web sites that either promise miracles or detail the end that awaits. I recognize now that I was putting off thinking about what was going to happen. I tried to concentrate on the few things I knew I had to do. This focusing helped me to cope in those first two months of treatment.

The issue of death was there, just below the surface, but I pushed it aside. There was too much else to do. Eventually I would begin to think more directly about what the future held for me, to think consciously about death.

4

The Initial Treatment

In truth, Michael's treatment regimen is not the standard, and by no means is it the appropriate initial treatment for the majority of patients with a new diagnosis of advanced pancreatic cancer. In fact, most patients with pancreatic cancer are initially treated with either gemcitabine alone or gemcitabine with one other agent. Our decision to start Michael on GTX mostly resulted from a variety of circumstances. I have some reservation that his story may be misinterpreted by patients or their families to mean that GTX should be their initial treatment.

My usual approach to discussing treatment options with a patient is to outline the following: (a) standard treatment options driven by "evidence-based medicine" or clinical trial data, (b) available current clinical trials, (c) known but not rigorously proven therapies, and (d) symptom management without "anticancer" therapy. The last option is often referred to as palliative care, but in reality, all of the treatment options for metastatic pancreatic cancer are palliative, based on the definition that to palliate a disease is to treat it partially but not cure it completely.

At any point in time, details of the treatment options will be outdated, because of emerging clinical trial data, but the underlying principles on which the treatment options are based remain the same. Indeed, I hope that details of various options will have changed by the time this chapter is read, for this would indicate that we have made progress in the treatment of patients with pancreatic cancer.

Gemcitabine was approved by the Food and Drug Administration (FDA) for the treatment of metastatic pancreatic cancer on the basis of a study, published over a decade ago in the *Journal of Clinical Oncology*, which reported a modest survival benefit (more people lived longer) and a significant clinical benefit (more people felt better) for those treated with gemcitabine than with another drug.[1] The median survival times were 5.65 months in the gemcitabine-treated group compared to 4.41 months in the group treated with 5-fluorouracil (5-FU). While this may not sound like a significant survival benefit, the percentage who survived at least 12 months was 18 percent versus 2 percent, respectively. An important observation was made during the initial trials with gemcitabine: a surprising percentage of patients, relative to the percentage whose tumors shrank, appeared also to benefit symptomatically from the chemotherapy. The percentage who had shrinkage of tumors, which is the "response rate" that studies are usually most concerned with, is actually only in the single digits. But as a result of this additional observation, this study reported a "clinical benefit response rate," which is a composite of symptomatic measures that include changes in pain, weight, and functional status. Clinical benefit was experienced by 23.8 percent of gemcitabine-treated patients compared with only 4.8 percent of 5-FU-treated patients.

I present these statistics not to be technical but to illustrate a couple of points. The first is that for this particular drug, gemcitabine, focusing on quality-of-life measures and "stable disease" was just as critical as focusing on traditional medical goals such as response rate and survival, in this highly symptomatic disease. The second point is that, while gemcitabine may not be appropriate for every newly diagnosed pancreatic cancer patient, understanding its history may help alleviate the fear often associated with chemotherapy. There are numerous chemotherapeutic agents, and they have different effects in different people. Hair loss is not common, and some patients actually feel better on chemotherapy.

There are many treatment options supported by clinical trials that include a combination of gemcitabine with a second agent. I also discussed these with Michael and Beth. The details of these combinations change with time, but the second agent is usually either a "targeted agent" or a second chemotherapeutic drug. While chemotherapy drugs also have targets, in oncology speak, targeted agents typically are substances that are known to seek out certain molecules that are believed to play a role in cancer progression.

One targeted agent that deserves mention, as it is FDA approved for pancreatic cancer, is the drug erlotinib, which targets human epidermal growth factor receptor type 1 (HER1/EGFR). In pancreatic tumors there is often too much of this growth factor receptor.[2] Growth factor receptors are proteins that sit on the surface of cells and send signals to the cell to grow and divide (see Figure 4.1). Erlotinib is an oral drug that is taken once a day every day during treatment. Taking erlotinib with gemcitabine, compared to gemcitabine alone, provides a modest improvement in median survival time (6.24 vs. 5.91 months). The percentage of patients who survive at least a year becomes 23 percent, versus 17 percent. This translates to an 18 percent reduction in the risk of death. While there are additional toxicities—erlotinib causes side effects—they are mostly mild to moderate. When I discuss with patients the option of adding erlotinib, I explain that a small percentage of patients will have a survival benefit from the combination but with some added toxicity. The decision to add erlotinib or not is made on a case-by-case basis and depends on patient and physician preferences.

Gemcitabine has been combined with a variety of other chemotherapeutic agents. In general, multiagent regimens have resulted in higher response rates—greater tumor shrinkage—but not in a

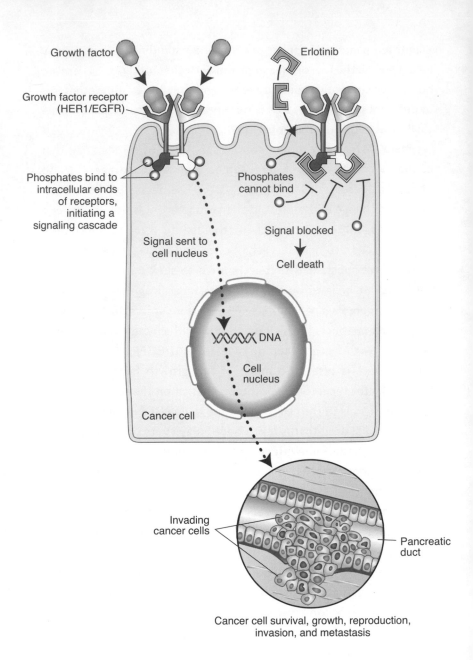

Figure 4.1 Erlotinib (Tarceva) works by blocking growth signals from growth factor receptors on the cancer cell's surface. This results in cell death and impairs growth and development of invasive tumors.

survival benefit. There are many reasons why a higher response rate might not result in improved survival. Response rates are determined by measurement of tumors on scans, and sometimes results can be biased by the investigator. Multiagent therapy may increase toxicity, which may ultimately affect survival. Theoretically, combination therapy could make a tumor more aggressive, so that the benefits of the initial response are obscured.

Also, tumor shrinkage that is short-lived is unlikely to improve overall survival. Many small pancreatic cancer trials have shown survival benefits that were not borne out in larger more rigorously designed multi-institutional studies. However, combination therapies, such as gemcitabine and capecitabine (Xeloda) or gemcitabine and a platinum (cisplatin or oxaliplatin), are often offered because improvement in survival has been shown in meta-analyses or subset analyses of good-performance-status patients.[3] A *meta-analysis* combines the results of several studies that address related research hypotheses or questions. *Performance status* refers to the level of activity of which a patient is capable; it indicates the impact of the cancer on the patient's ability to perform regular daily activities.

A large study from France has recently been reported in abstract form at the American Society of Clinical Oncology 2010 meeting. It demonstrated that FOLFIRINOX (5-fluorouracil, leucovorin, irinotecan, and oxaliplatin) resulted in an overall survival of 10.4 months, compared with 6.8 months with gemcitabine alone. This regimen should be reserved for patients with near normal bilirubin levels and good performance status. Enthusiasm for this regimen is tempered by the rate of negative side effects: peripheral neuropathy (damage to nerves), hair loss, neutropenia (low white blood cell count), and fatigue. While I am open to using this regimen, I will do so with caution, given concerns for potential side effects.[4]

Great care must be taken in translating clinical trial data to everyday clinical practice. The eligibility criteria to enter most studies include a good performance status, so studies tend to involve patients who are stronger. In addition, patients have to have adequate kidney, liver, and bone marrow function to participate in most trials. Patients who meet clinical trial eligibility are not necessarily the types of patients we see in our office every day.

CHOOSING THE APPROPRIATE THERAPY

This leads me to skip to the last therapeutic option Michael listed in Chapter 3 and that is "to do nothing." Technically, this option is not "to do nothing" but to focus on palliation without the use of conventional chemotherapy. One of the tenets of medicine is to "first do no harm," and one of the tenets of oncology is to not use chemotherapy if a patient has a poor "performance status." Patients' performance status at the time of diagnosis is an indicator of both their prognosis and how they are likely to respond to treatment. Chemotherapy is often not prescribed for patients with poor performance status because these patients are unlikely to benefit from it and more likely to suffer from toxicity.

Patients who might be able to tolerate treatment may also choose not to embark on a path that includes chemotherapy, feeling that the modest potential benefit will not be worth the energy and time or the perceived risks. Therefore, the options presented to a particular patient have to be tailored to that individual's circumstances. At times, palliative care is the most appropriate option. In truth, it can be difficult for a physician to present this option, for fear of a negative reaction from the patient and his family. This is especially true when they have traveled to "the great Johns Hopkins Hospital" for a second opinion.

From my own experience, it is only the frail elderly or patients who have not tolerated prior chemotherapeutic interventions well who understand and accept the palliative therapy option without some amount of convincing. A typical response is "we should try something," but doing "something" is not always better than doing "nothing." In fact, some palliative care literature suggests that some individuals who choose hospice care over "active" treatment have a survival advantage, that is, they live longer than those who get more assertive treatment. There are probably many reasons for this longer survival, including less toxicity from therapies and more comprehensive symptom and psychosocial intervention.

Michael and Beth did not strike me as people who would consider no chemotherapy, at least at this point in their journey. He had previously been feeling well and his performance status was well preserved.

This brings us to the two middle options that I typically present to patients: clinical trial participation and known but not rigorously proven therapies. I practice oncology in an academic medical center, and part of being at a research institution is promoting clinical trial participation when a patient might be appropriate for a clinical study. This is not to say that clinical research is restricted to academic centers, and in truth, much of clinical trial recruitment is performed out in community medical practices. Pancreatic cancer is a disease with limited treatment options and few successes. While giving good care to our patients comes first, our goal is also to learn as much as possible from patients who are appropriate for clinical trials. In doing so, we might gain insight with which to help future patients who will be diagnosed with this disease.

A typical pancreatic cancer study combines a new agent with gemcitabine. The patient gets a component of standard-of-care treatment while receiving an additional agent that we hope will improve the treatment outcome. At the time of Michael's consultation, we had only one trial open, and that study would not be accepting patients for a few weeks, and then the enrollment process might take a while. I am sure that patients who have participated or tried to participate in a clinical trial have experienced some of the frustration with the timing required to actually enroll in a trial. Waiting to begin treatment did not seem appropriate in Michael's case.

The open trial involved an agent in the class of drugs referred to as "taxanes." The treatment option I then presented to Michael, a combination of gemcitabine, Taxotere, and Xeloda (GTX), also includes a taxane, Taxotere. I had recently read more about GTX, as a number of patients had come to me in consultation asking about this regimen. Additionally, one patient had told me about his unexpectedly good response to the regimen. As a relative newcomer to oncology, I feel somewhat obligated to make a cautionary note before I describe this regimen further. Many patients do not tolerate or respond to combination chemotherapy as well as Michael, and some physicians might disapprove that this regimen was offered outside the context of a clinical trial, given that there is limited published data supporting its use. But the truth is that when treatment options and research data are very limited, sometimes physicians, for good or for bad, can be influenced by the anecdotal evidence of patient experiences.

Robert Fine and his colleagues at Columbia University developed this GTX regimen based on their laboratory observations that the combination of these drugs, given together and in a particular sequence, had a synergistic effect on the death of cancer cells in a culture dish.[5] The gemcitabine is given over a prolonged period by infusion (intravenously); Margaret Tempero and her colleagues at the University of California, San Francisco showed that gemcitabine works better given by this method. A retrospective review of 35 patients treated with GTX a few years earlier was reported in 2007 and showed an 11.2-month median survival, a 43 percent 12-month survival, and an 11 percent 30-month survival. However, these data are not considered rigorous, as the report is on only 35 patients and the data is retrospective, meaning that the study looked at past events. This type of study does not control for the inherent biases, such as the selection of patients who are more likely to do well and differences in the supportive care given the patients. Prospective studies, which are studies that look forward in time, eliminate some bias, because the investigators do not know the outcome until the study ends. A small, prospective study of 35 patients demonstrated a median survival of 14.5 months.[6] Since the time of these publications, it is likely that hundreds of patients have been treated with this regimen, both on protocols by the Columbia group and "off protocol," which means not in the context of a clinical trial. Unfortunately, when patients are treated off protocol, it is difficult to collect information on patient characteristics, response, survival, and toxicity. This information is critical to making a treatment option "generalizable" to other patients.

My recollection of that consultation with Michael and Beth is that, even though Beth was vigorously taking notes, they were too stunned by the diagnosis to make a treatment decision at that moment. It was a "you're the doctor, you tell us what to do" moment. I tried to follow their cues regarding their preferences. My sense was that they wanted therapy and did not want to try gemcitabine alone. So, despite the limited data, we opted to start treatment with GTX.

The pretreatment evaluation and consultation provides the physician an opportunity to assess whether or not the patient is appropriate for therapy. The medical history and physical exam are supplemented with laboratory studies to help in the decision whether to initiate treatment and how to monitor treatment. One of the most important purposes of the history and physical is to determine the patient's functional status. A person with multiple medical problems or moderate to severe limitations in functional status is less likely to do well with or without treatment. Michael did not fit this category. While he had symptoms of abdominal pain and weight loss, these were not particularly limiting. His medical history did not include any diagnoses that made treatment with any of the agents we were considering particularly dangerous.

Laboratory tests were done to assess kidney, liver, and bone marrow function. The kidneys and liver are assessed before treatment to establish a baseline, and they are monitored throughout the course of therapy for several reasons. These organs are necessary for the proper metabolism of the chemotherapy drugs, and the doses may have to be adjusted or eliminated depending on the status of these two organs. Ongoing monitoring can also provide clues of either damage from the chemotherapy or the development of other conditions, such as dehydration or progression of liver metastases. Bone marrow function is also critical to follow, as chemotherapy particularly affects cell division, such as that which happens in the bone marrow. This is monitored by a complete blood count (CBC) or a hematology profile (heme-8). The hemoglobin or hematocrit tells us if the patient is developing anemia and may need a blood transfusion. The platelet count tells us if the patient may be at increased risk for bleeding and whether the dose of drugs has to be reduced or withheld.

Most importantly, the white blood cell count, and in particular the neutrophil count, tells us if the patient is at increased risk for infection and may need urgent antibiotics if he develops a fever. A drop in neutrophil count is particularly important, as life threatening consequences could result if antibiotics are not started quickly in someone with what we refer to as a neutropenic fever, which is a fever in someone with a low neutrophil count.

Other side effects that patients can experience on chemotherapy are changes in taste, decreased appetite, decreased energy, diarrhea, constipation, mouth sores, nausea, and vomiting. These side effects are common to a number of drugs. The newer supportive drugs for treatment of chemotherapy-associated nausea, while they do not work for everyone, are much more effective than the previous generation of such medications.

Another critical assessment before the initiation of care is the patient's social supports. Michael had Beth at his side at the initial consultation, so my assumption was that she would be his support. This is a huge responsibility and requires a great deal of patience and stamina. Once treatment started, Michael had to get used to essentially being a patient almost on a daily basis, as much of his life revolved around getting to and from treatments and worrying about the side effects in between the visits. I have to admit that, after an initial consultation that lasts only an hour, I have not always adequately assessed a patient's social situation before initiating therapy.

In other cases, I have learned the hard way that a patient will miss an appointment because of lack of child care or the fear of losing his job and its benefits. Patients' lives are complex.

PAIN MANAGEMENT

Another issue we address on an ongoing basis is pain control. Patients fear the unknown, they fear death, and they fear pain. Oncologists do not have any magical ways to alleviate these fears, but we do have access to effective therapies for the alleviation of pain. In general, cancer pain is undertreated. There are guidelines for the treatment of adult cancer pain, and they are available to all physicians.[7] An important component of these guidelines is regular reassessment, to ensure that the pain intervention is having the desired effect. Pain management often rises in steps, from agents such as acetaminophen (Tylenol) and nonsteroidal anti-inflammatory agents such as ibuprofen (Motrin or Advil) to a "weak opioid" such as codeine and then to a "strong opioid" such as morphine. For most patients with pancreatic cancer, the non-opioid medications by themselves provide insufficient management of pain. Patients with cancer also have to be careful when using acetaminophen and/or ibuprofen, because these agents can mask a fever or infection, and over time they can damage the liver and kidneys. Typically, I start with a short-acting opioid such as morphine or oxycodone, to be used as needed. If a pattern of frequent use is established, a long-acting opioid can be selected in the right dose, so that there is a slow release of an analgesic to provide constant pain control. The short-acting drugs are then used for what we refer to as break-through pain. Patients usually need to take stool softeners and often laxatives when starting opioids, as constipation is a common side effect. Since Michael's pain was relatively constant, we opted to start with a low dose of a long-acting opioid taken orally every 12 hours.

In addition to pain, there are many other issues that may need to be addressed in an initial consultation, such as depression, advanced directives, and nutrition. There is a very limited amount of time in the initial interview, and some level of rapport is often necessary before discussion of some of these topics. While physicians should be responsible for touching on some of these areas with patients, one of the benefits of working in a cancer center is access to a palliative care team, social workers, and dieticians to help address the other issues encountered along a patient's journey.

5

The Prospect of Death

DOING WHAT HAS TO BE DONE

As I started chemotherapy, I put off thinking about death. I focused my thoughts on what I believed I could control. I assumed I was dying.

Putting My Affairs in Order

During those first two months, my goal was to do what had to be done. My training as a lawyer channeled my thinking. I liked to think I was logical, even if I sometimes suffered terrible lapses in logic. The first thing I thought about was my final will. I was determined to draft a new one.

I remember how much time I spent trying to figure out what to do with my modest assets. It was *so* calming. This might not work for everyone, but it did help me. I spent days figuring out what to give to whom. Three of my four sons live overseas. There were tax questions. There were lists of credit cards that would need to be canceled, and banks and insurance companies that would need to be notified. There were questions concerning the executor. All of this occupied my mind from morning to night, and helped me to get to sleep. I became obsessed with trying to tie up all the loose ends.

When I retired from the federal government, I had made certain choices concerning my life insurance that I now wished to change. I could do this because I had not yet turned 65. Nevertheless, it was complicated and eventually meant arguing with some parts of the governmental bureaucracy. Finally, I was successful. I was also helped by that same bureaucracy.

I worried about who would be the executor of my estate. Beth refused this job, probably for good reasons. I finally decided to name my local bank as the executor. It would be more expensive than having Beth or one of my sons do it, but some of the stories I had read about the problems that can happen when one family member, among many, is the executor, convinced me that a bank was the right way to go. It may save a lot of grief.

One of the most helpful books on this subject that I found had the rather somber title *Beyond the Grave: The Right Way and the Wrong Way of Leaving Money to Your Children (and Others).*[1] I read and reread it. It consistently and strongly advised using a bank as executor.

Through all of this, during those first two months, Beth and I didn't talk very much about what death might be or mean. What it would be like to die. It was there. I expected it, but I was not ready to think about it. It was more important that I leave with as little unfinished business as possible. I wanted to be like Jane Brody's Anna Engquist, who had everything carefully ordered before she went into surgery. Still, what drove all this was the expectation, unspoken mostly, that I was going to die soon.

First reactions to a cancer diagnosis vary considerably from person to person, of course. As time went on and I was able to read more and to talk to others about their first reactions, I came to think that my reactions had been normal. First there is shock, then there is numbness.

A friend told me a similar story.[2] During a regular mammogram, the radiologist noticed something out of the ordinary. A biopsy was scheduled. Before the biopsy, her doctor told her that he did not think the irregularity was malignant. He had rarely been wrong on these assessments. She was so confident that the results of the biopsy were going to be okay that she did not ask anyone to go with her to her meeting with the doctor. She drove to the appointment by herself. Alas, her doctor delivered bad news. She had breast cancer. She was shocked, so shocked she had great difficulty focusing on what the doctor was saying. Her shock turned to numbness. She wished with all her heart that she had had someone with her.

Focusing on doing what had to be done allowed me not to dwell on the longer-term future, such as it might be. That seemed to be the way many people manage. Whether it is putting your affairs in order, or doing as Anna Engquist did, putting her house in order and telling her friends and family goodbye, with love, each person finds his or her own way of coping. It may be something as simple as wanting to have family and friends around. There is not a single way to do this. It is a very personal journey.

One older woman I was told about came home from her diagnosis of terminal cancer and sat down and composed a long and heartfelt letter that she sent out to her family and friends, telling them the news. This was the most important thing for her, something only she could do, and something that she spent considerable time composing in order to say exactly what she felt to those she loved.[3]

Tasks and Goals

Much of what was going to happen would be out of my control. However, there were things I could control, and I think that for everyone these things should be the focus during the first weeks after diagnosis. At this point in the journey, one needs tasks more than goals.

Having goals is different from concentrating on things that can be controlled and that have to be done. Goals come a little later. Longer-term goals can instill some hope for the future. Living long enough to attend my granddaughter's graduation from high school was one that I had. She lives in Philadelphia and we had attended most of the important events in her life, including birthdays and graduations. We were so proud when we attended her high school graduation in June 2009.

Voting in the next presidential election was another goal. I remember telling Dr. Le that it was very important to me to stick around long enough to vote in November 2008. Of course, she could not promise this, but it became a real goal.

These kinds of goals give your body and mind something to fasten onto, and to look forward to.

Another goal, which I will talk more about in Chapter 7, concerned my desire to have a new car. Although we certainly did not need another car, I leased a VW beetle convertible in April 2008. It was a thirty-month lease. I wanted to have the full value of that lease. I told everyone I was determined to live until the end of the lease, at least thirty more months.

Reviewing Legal Documents

But I'm getting ahead of myself. The immediate tasks within my control were putting my affairs in order: my will, my living will or advance health directives, designation of a health proxy, and my life insurance.

I had each of these, but I needed to look at them again. They were not old, but they were already out-of-date. Much had happened since I'd drawn them up. There were more grandchildren and different assets. I also had to review the disposition of assets outside of the will and bring these up to date. Such things as mutual funds, life insurance, and real property can often be passed upon your death to others outside a formal will, so it is important to review the status of these matters as well.

The living will and the health proxy required additional work. A living will tells the world, but more importantly health care providers, family, and the legal system, what should happen if you are unable to tell them directly because of being unconscious or in a coma.

The health proxy is different. It gives legal authority to a designated person to make health care decisions in the event that the designating person is unable to do so. I was not quite sure what would happen in the event of a conflict between the two documents (I believe the written instructions take precedence). It would likely depend on state law, but I knew it was important that Beth, my proxy, understand what I wanted. We went over the health proxy document in detail. I am very comfortable that she will act as I request.

One thing to remember is to have these instructions available. They are not of any use if health care providers and family do not know their contents or where they are.

For people with dependent children, there are any number of excellent articles and books that advise on this subject. But even for those of us who are older, these documents should not be neglected.

Some people may be reluctant to face these issues. I was not one of those people. This was something I needed to do. Really, I think I just fastened onto it as something I could do myself. If I had not had that, I am not sure what would have happened. I called my attorney within a week of my diagnosis and we agreed on a plan to draft a final will.

Earlier I mentioned the living will. Jane Brody, in her excellent *Guide to the Great Beyond*,[4] also wrote of the importance of making sure that the instructions in the living will about near-to-death situations are as clear as possible. One reason to do this is that the process of keeping someone alive in an emergency can be harrowing. Many times, it is physically painful, yet unsuccessful.[5]

My guess is that, if I did not have a living will, if I had not really thought about it and talked it over with Beth, if no one knew my wishes, my family would want to do everything possible to save my life in an emergency situation. If that is not your desired goal, you must make it known.

As I did research for this book, I found this area of dying wishes to be complicated and murky. Each state has different requirements. Like a will, the advance directives need to be tailored to a particular state's legal requirements. At the same time, they must be general enough to be applicable in other states, should the need arise. As with many things, it is important to consult a good attorney when creating a legal document, if possible.

Having clear, detailed instructions about what you wish done when death approaches, whether by long-term illness or accident or sudden illness, is important for at least two reasons.

First, when the end is near, one might not want to be kept alive artificially by the many means that modern medicine has at its disposal these days. It is one thing to be dying peacefully under hospice care, where everyone knows exactly what is to be done. It is quite another to be in a strange place, unknown, at a hospital that might be legally obligated to take all possible measures, when that is the last thing desired by you and your family.

The second reason for being clear is exactly the opposite. You may wish to be revived even if there is a cancer that is going to kill you eventually. Suppose there is an emergency, from whatever cause. Suppose it is possible to be saved, *and still be in reasonably good condition mentally and physically afterwards*, even if it means living for only another few months, and that is your desire. The last thing you want is to have someone decide, because there is a "do not resuscitate" or "do not take extraordinary measures" note somewhere, that no further efforts should be made to keep you alive.

Not only is it important to have clear directives, it is crucial that these directives be known and the written document available. Otherwise, the hospital's hands may be tied. This almost happened in one case of a woman who had had a stroke. As her condition deteriorated, everyone in the family knew that she was dying and that she did not want to live on a feeding tube. She had written these instructions down earlier, but the paper was in her safe-deposit box at the bank. It was a holiday and the bank was closed. The written instructions could not be retrieved, and the doctors and hospital were worried about the looming legal situation. Without a living will or a health care power-of-attorney or proxy designation, the doctors told the family, the hospital would be obligated to take extra-ordinary measures to save her life if she got any worse. Luckily, she survived the night, and the next day the family was able to get the documents, avoid the extraordinary measures, and have her trans-ferred to a hospice facility where she could die naturally.[6]

We need to be careful here. Although in many cases families are told that hospitals are required, in the absence of documentation instructing otherwise, to try to keep patients alive, doctors opt not to use extraordinary measures all the time based only on what the family says are the patient's wishes, even without the physical paper in hand. Of course, there is also the other side of the coin, that it is better to be safe than sorry.

You can see why it is important that instructions be written, known, and available. Although not all the possible situations in the world can be covered by advance directives, there is much that can be clarified.

Ms. Brody provides an excellent discussion and offers examples of these issues in the chapter about advance directives in her book.[7] There are also models available on the Internet. After seeing these, I decided to change my advance directives. I made an extensive and explicit list of procedures I did not want, such as a ventilator, intu-bation, and defibrillation.

I also included one additional section, an exceptions clause that allows Beth (and Beth alone) to overrule what I have directed, under the specific circumstance that medical opinion agrees that specific emergency measures would allow me to resume a life of reasonable quality for a period of time. This is my effort to have one last chance to do something I want, if possible.

OTHER FUNDAMENTAL ISSUES

Six weeks after diagnosis, toward the end of January 2008, my initial focus on immediate concerns began to shift. It became clear that it was time to face up to the issue of death itself.

This is a solitary journey. It is also frightening. Most friends and family will not want to talk with you about death, out of concern for you, and in fact, they will not know how to do it. They will likely be uncomfortable. This is understandable. There are people who are trained to talk about death, who can be consulted to help with this process. Other patients with pancreatic or other cancers also may not feel able or wish to discuss this with you. It is not a subject that comes up in the chemo pod. Although I knew what was happening to many of us, and they knew, it was still impossible to talk directly about feelings as death approached.

Understanding the Physical Process of Dying

My own thoughts turned increasingly toward the dying process. I began to think about it every night. What was uppermost in my mind was trying to understand how death would come and what it would feel like. I was most concerned about what would happen physically. I wondered what it would be like as the cancer spread and I grew weaker.

A month after my diagnosis, in early January 2008, Beth and I drove down to visit her family in North Carolina. Beth goes for treatment for migraine headaches in Chicago once a quarter but had been unable to make the trip in December because of my illness; I was not able to be alone at that time. Beth's family was very willing to help look out for me if we came to North Carolina. They had been good to me since our first meeting six years before, and I felt at home there. We usually went to see them for Christmas, but because of the diagnosis, and because I was just beginning treatment, we had not gone for Christmas 2007. It seemed like a good idea for us to go and for Beth to make up her missed appointment. Beth could fly to Chicago and I would stay with my mother-in-law. Beth's sister Nan and her husband Tom live next door, so there would be additional help if needed.

Everything went well. The trip down was smooth. We packed the back seat of the car with doggy pillows. I could lie down very comfortably and I could raise my head to look out. When I raised my head, I felt like a little dog perched in the back seat and looking out the open window, eager to see what was happening.

Once we arrived, I was installed on the second floor of the house, from which I rarely ventured. I was too tired to go downstairs. Beth's mother, bless her, brought food up the stairs to me in a basket. She would hold the rail to climb the stairs in order to balance the weight of the basket.

While down in North Carolina I had a long conversation with a friend about what death might be like. She recommended that I read Dr. Raymond A. Moody's book about near-death experiences, *Life after Life*.[8] I read with great fascination the description of people who had gone to the brink of death, reported seeing a great white light, or other manifestations, but then came back to tell about it.

I am not a religious person. I have never believed in life after death, even as a child. But, to be honest, I had never pursued the matter. I had gotten as far as thinking that the idea of life after death is comforting to some people, and if so, that is fine for them. And so it was with my response to *Life after Life*. I could not really believe in it. I wanted more proof, more concrete answers.

Many people have faith in God and truly believe in a life hereafter. This is the case with a friend of ours who has had two kinds of breast cancer, seven years apart. Her faith is strong, and this helps her to face what might happen. She tells me that something very special is happening with me, and this has certainly comforted me, even if I cannot quite attribute it to the hand of God.

I have to admit, however, that my habit of trying to cover all bases persists. On a recent trip to Mexico, I discovered the story of Saint Charbel, the patron saint of lost causes, at least in Oaxaca. I decided to buy a small figure of him, and he now sits securely in my bedroom, watching over me, I hope.

Beth was able to help with some of this. She knew someone who had died in an in-house hospice care program. Although he had not died from cancer, his illness was serious and his time in the hospice had gone well. This was reassuring.

What preoccupied me most was pain at the end of life. I needed to understand the process of dying, physiologically. I began to read more. I found Sherwin Nuland's book *How We Die*[9] to be the most helpful. It describes in great detail how the body shuts down as life comes to an end.

This process takes place with all extended illnesses, not just cancer. The book is explicit and thorough. It talks about seven major illnesses. It is helpful in explaining what cancer is and how it acts on the body's various systems. Of course, I was primarily interested in cancer and Dr. Nuland wrote very clearly about what cancer is. This helped me to understand what might happen. He wrote, in part:

> Cancer is best viewed as a disease of altered maturation; it is the result of a multistage process of growth and development having gone awry. Under ordinary conditions, normal cells are constantly being replaced as they die . . . As they get closer to full maturity, they lose their ability to proliferate rapidly in proportion to their ability to perform the functions for which they are intended as grown-ups. A fully mature cell of the intestinal lining, for example, absorbs nutriments from the cavity of the gut a lot more efficiently than it reproduces; a fully mature thyroid cell is at its best when it secretes hormone, but it is less inclined to reproduce than it was while younger . . . A tumor cell is one that has somewhere along the way been stopped in its capacity to differentiate, which is the term used by scientists for the process by which cells go through the steps that enable them to reach healthy adulthood. The clump of immature abnormal cells that results from the blocking of differentiation is called a neoplasm . . . used synonymously with tumor. Those tumors whose cells have been blocked closest to the attainment of the mature state are the least dangerous and are therefore called benign. A benign tumor has retained relatively little of its potential for uncontrolled reproduction—it is well differentiated; under the microscope, it looks a lot like the adult it was close to becoming. It grows slowly, does not invade surrounding tissues or travel to other

parts of the body, is often surrounded by a distinct fibrous capsule, and almost never has the capacity to kill its host . . . A malignant neoplasm—what we call cancer—is a different creature entirely. Some influence or combination of influences, whether genetic, environmental, or otherwise, has acted as the triggering mechanism to interfere so early in the pathway of maturation that the progress of the cells has been stopped at a stage when they still have an infinite capacity to reproduce.[10]

It is well and good to understand this, but I discovered that what I wanted to know, what I needed to know, was not only how death happens but also what it is going to feel like, physically, to die. I was afraid, and I felt that knowing more would make me less afraid.

I asked Dr. Le, in general terms, about death. She suggested I talk with someone on her team about this. A social worker came to see me the next time I was having chemo.

At first, she did not understand what I was looking for. She talked about hospice care. Finally, I was able to make her understand that I needed to know what would happen to me physically, what I would feel. As I said this, I realized that what I was seeking was reassurance that the end would be peaceful and painless. She could not tell me that, but she was able to make me understand that everything that could be done would be done to make it a painless passing. When I understood this, I was able to calm down.

I felt I knew what was coming. It was not that I was in control, but at least I was not going to be surprised.

For someone with a long-lasting disease, the end comes as various organs in the body begin to shut down. There are many different possible symptoms. I hope the path I take is to feel less and less like eating until I finally stop taking solid food. I want to take liquids, but toward the end I will probably lose this desire as well. If there is pain, as is likely as the cancer spreads, this pain can most likely be managed. I will sleep much more. Gradually, I will slip into unconsciousness. And then be no more.

This is what I needed to know and what I needed to believe. It comforted me to know that death could happen this way.

As I write this, more than two years later, I can only shake my head. There is no way that one can ever really know how death will come and whether it is going to be painful, and if the pain can be controlled. However, I was ready to believe that. I wanted to believe it. And once I believed, the issue was behind me.

I do not mean to say that I no longer fear death. This was brought home recently in a conversation I had with Dr. Le and Beth concerning autopsies. My heart started beating rapidly and I realized how difficult it still is to admit to myself and accept that this is really going to happen. I think I will never lose my fear of death. I can accept the inevitable in my mind but not in my heart.

Grief and Anger

One of the books I skimmed during my research into death was Elisabeth Kübler-Ross's *On Death and Dying*, published in 1969.[11] She had worked with terminally ill people in Chicago. She believed that it was better to talk about death with those who were dying, to hear what they had to say, and to understand what they were feeling, a way of doing things that was not common in the 1960s. From her research emerged descriptions of the five major stages of grief, which most people experience in some way after being diagnosed with a terminal illness. These stages are denial, anger, bargaining, depression, and acceptance.

Remembering these stages is helpful in many ways for understanding what is happening when one is terminally ill, even if those dying do not go through the stages in exactly the same way. I tried to think about my own experience. I really could not figure out whether I had gone through these stages at all. I never actually denied what was happening. For me, death became a given. But then again, perhaps focusing on revising all my documents had been a form of denial. I do not think I bargained. I was certainly depressed at times, and I was given a medication for depression that seems to work. I credit it with making me less argumentative.

I did not experience anger in the sense that I was angry at being singled out and did not understand why. For a while, I thought that I had accepted my fate, though I always had hope I would live a bit longer. In a way, this is denial, but it did not seem that way to me at the time.

Then things began to happen that made me realize I was angry underneath, in my own particular, perhaps peculiar, way. I bring this situation up at this point, even though I am not proud of it, but this happens to people with a terminal illness, and people should not be surprised by it.

In the first few months after my diagnosis, I thought that because I was dying I should pretty much have my way in everything. In fact, this was not unusual for me. I have always liked to have my own way, although I had been perhaps less overt about it in the past.

While deferring to me in many things, Beth did not agree with all my desires. Some of the things I wanted were impossible in our situation, she pointed out, or were putting her in a position of having more to do than she could handle. This was the case with our property. It required considerable care and constant attention and was a responsibility she took very seriously.

For some reason, most likely from a sense that I had to be right, that I was entitled to be right, I took Beth's protests to mean that she was not concerned for me and was already planning what she would do after I was gone. At times I believed that she was angry for allowing herself to remain in a sometimes-rocky marriage, only to find herself tied to me now. I tried to make her admit this; it made sense to me. After all, she would be free of me and would be alive after I was gone.

At other times, more rationally, I saw Beth as a victim. We had been married only five years and we had hopes and dreams like many retired people to travel and see the world. When we married, we had both counted on growing old together. I felt bad for her that this was not to be.

However, more often than not, my feelings about my coming death and my immediate desires outweighed my concern for her.

Finally, later, I began to admit to myself that her concern for me was genuine. She believed deeply in the vows she had made. However, it took her persistent care in the face of my rejection and anger to make me realize this. One incident helped bring this home to me. As I mentioned in Chapter 3, in June 2008 I had to go to the ER with a fever. Because my immune system was compromised by the chemotherapy, I was under instructions to go to an emergency room immediately if I developed a high fever. We had to go in a rush; my temperature had risen quickly. Beth took charge and drove us there, and she remained with me for the six long hours it took to get everything sorted out at the hospital. Of course, this is not an exceptional thing for a spouse to do. She had always stayed with me in the chemo pod and had taken me everywhere I needed to go. Somehow, that day, my thinking changed. It finally penetrated. I began to believe that Beth did care and that I was wrong to doubt her motives.

My difficulty in accepting her care showed that I had not accepted what was happening. I had been angry with Beth on a deeply emotional level for continuing to live when I could not.

I was not yet prepared to die, I was still hopeful that I might have more time. Prepare for the worst and hope for the best, as Dr. Le says. I try to follow this. I have put my affairs in order and worked to understand how death might happen. That is as far as I can go at this point in preparing for the worst.

Hoping for the best meant different things to me at different times. Early on, it meant hoping for a little extra time to be in this world. As time passed, hoping for the best began to mean thinking about other things I might do while still alive. I had not really considered "the value" of my life to others. I was 64. I thought I had had a pretty good life. I believed I had contributed some good to the world. I did not think longer term. Later on, I began to think about ways I might be able to continue to do some good in the world before I left, with my family and perhaps more broadly.

I still have a feeling in the pit of my stomach when I think about my coming death. I believe most people accept the inevitable. After all, it is the inevitable. Those who are religious may more easily accept it. Those who are not may still give thanks for having led a life of value. I expect everyone comes to acceptance in his or her own way, with some kind of grace. I believe the secret lies in becoming more aware, as I try to, of what is so frightening about death.

While all of this was going on, much of it simultaneously in those early months of 2008, family and friends were asking to be admitted to our world. However, as with everything else, this proved not to be easy.

6

Balancing Hope and Truth

ADVANCE HEALTH CARE DIRECTIVES

Given the time constraints, it is not uncommon for a physician with a waiting room full of patients to get wrapped up in the details of treatments, side effects, and symptom management and not to have time to discuss other important issues. Conversations regarding subjects such as death and advance directives often are postponed until pushed to the forefront by a medical crisis. Advance directives are legal documents that allow patients to convey their choices about health care, and, as the term suggests, they are meant to be done in advance. During a crisis, it is difficult to proceed in a manner consistent with the patient's wishes if the patient's preferences have not been previously outlined to the family or the physician, preferably in writing. Commonly, doctors are not aware whether or not a patient has drawn up advance directives. Ironically, it was only when reviewing Michael's chapters for this book that I learned that he has advance directives in place.

Having your wishes in writing increases the chance that they will be carried out if you are unable to communicate your wishes. At a minimum, your wishes should be communicated to your family, so that there is no confusion regarding your intentions, especially in regards to end-of-life decisions. Two good resources for exploring these issues are the oncology social worker and Web sites such as Aging with Dignity and Caring Information.[1] The Web site covers information relevant to each state in the country, because regulations vary from state to state.

Advance directive documents include a living will, a durable power of attorney for health care, and a do-not-resuscitate (DNR) order. A living will is a document that describes the kinds of medical treatments you want or do not want in the event that you become incapacitated. It is not the same as a last will and testament, which is a legal declaration by which you name who will manage your estate and provide for the transfer of your assets upon death, and which can name a guardian for minor children. Patients are encouraged to speak with a lawyer if they want to create an actual will, outside of a living will or naming a health care proxy. Advance health care directives cover medical issues, not personal or financial. A durable power of attorney and a health care proxy document can make treatment decisions on your behalf if you are incapacitated. A DNR is a document that directs what measures should or should not be taken on your behalf in events such as a cardiac arrest (loss of a pulse) or respiratory arrest (loss of spontaneous breathing). Cardiopulmonary resuscitation (CPR) is a procedure used when a patient's heart stops beating and breathing stops, and it often involves rescue breathing, chest compressions, and electrical shocks to the heart. In many circumstances, it will be performed as a matter of course on a person whose heart and breathing have stopped, unless there is a do-not-resuscitate order in place.

Even when CPR is successful in reviving the person, it sometimes does not provide a significant extension of survival. In one study, done in a university teaching hospital, only 14 percent of patients who received CPR while hospitalized were discharged from the hospital.[2] The survival rate for resuscitated hospitalized patients with cancer is even lower. I am not trying to say that all patients with a cancer diagnosis should have a DNR order. This decision is often a difficult one, and an individual's particular circumstances play a crucial role. If circulation or breathing stop because of the relentless progression of the disease or a complication of progressive disease, doing chest compressions and mechanical ventilation are more likely to cause suffering than benefit. Just recently, when I was serving as the attending physician on the inpatient service, a decision about the removal of a ventilator had to be made in the case of a young woman with end-stage metastatic cancer. Her mother wanted to wait until her daughter woke up and could help make the decision. Unfortunately, it was not clear that the patient would wake up and be sound enough of mind to help make any decisions. From a physician's perspective, and probably from a caregiver's perspective, these emotional decisions are much easier if the patient and her family have discussed potential scenarios in advance. Sometimes a physician will get caught up in the emotional roller coaster of these difficult situations and unintentionally fuel the unrealistic hope that one more trial of therapy may have benefit for the patient. The physician's colleagues can see the reality more clearly from the sidelines.

HOW MUCH HOPE?

The practice of oncology would be simpler if the doctor-patient relationship were a science. A guiding formula that would define the proper balance between the infusion of hope and the description of reality would certainly be welcome when dealing with terminally ill patients. Oncology programs acknowledge the importance of this aspect of the job, and provide training with dedicated readings and role-playing activities, but there is no formula for empathy and the best way to deliver bad news. Articles in oncology journals try to provide practical advice on achieving a balance between honesty and hope. Eric Kodish, M.D., who is an oncologist and bioethicist, and Stephen Post, Ph.D., a bioethicist, stated it well in an article in the *Journal of Clinical Oncology:* "Doctors have a clear obligation to initiate discussions to inform patients about the diagnosis, specifics of treatment options and their side effects, and of the prognosis in general terms . . . But doctors must also respect patients' prerogative to decline further information, and should guard against exhaustive disclosure for the moral comfort of the physician, rather than the actual needs of the individual patient."[3]

Even in writing this book, I am concerned that the tone may be too direct and may discourage patients. But I think hearing Michael's story and perspective does provide a sense of hope. Providing a patient with hope does not mean resorting to deception or giving false hope. Implicit in the prescription of chemotherapy is the instillation of hope. Hope does not have to be for a cure or the prolongation of life. Realistic hope—as in Michael's case—may be for better symptom control, more strength to get one's affairs in order, participation in the election of the first African-American president, attendance at a graduation, or the completion of a book that will have impact on others. However, hope should not be provided at all costs, and there is a limit to what health care providers can accommodate, especially if that includes chemotherapy that they know will be ineffective and potentially harmful.

The *Journal of Clinical Oncology* periodically readdresses these issues in the series "The Art of Oncology: When the Tumor Is Not the Target." In one publication, two palliative care physicians, Jamie H. Von Roenn and Charles F. von Gunten, outline some practical guidelines for a therapeutic relationship: Establish that truth telling will be the norm unless the patient prefers otherwise. Prevent surprises by letting patients and families know that you are going to talk about all possible eventualities. Prepare for decision points in advance by telling them that you will let them know when you think the burden imposed by treatment exceeds the possible benefit.[4]

My personal style may be a little more direct than some patients might like, as I strive not to be the doctor who "never told me I was not curable." I think the reality is that in most cases, patients are told that they are not curable but they may not understand the implications of words such as "palliative." Certainly, patients may also suffer from some degree of denial or may have difficulty processing the overload of information given to them.

My experiences have softened my approach over time. While I think it is important to address prognosis early in the relationship, abrupt delivery of information can hinder the development of the patient's trust. Gauging what a patient is ready to hear has to be balanced with informing him of the known natural history of a disease. It may be counterintuitive, but I do feel some relief when a patient asks, "Dr. Le, how long do I have to live?" Of course, there is no exact answer for this question. Certainly, in Michael's case, he has already outlived the median survival time. But being asked this question does give me permission to address the important question of prognosis. I recall several episodes in my training and early faculty career that have left a lasting impression on me. There was a case of a young professional woman with small children who had had surgery for breast cancer and came to the oncology clinic to discuss treatment options to reduce the risk of recurrence. I assumed that she would want to know enough statistics to make an informed decision before undergoing therapy, so I started to pull up a Web-based program to obtain her numbers. She politely told me that she did not want to see the numbers and that she was ready to start therapy. She did not want to know her prognosis on that initial visit and she did not need to know the estimated magnitude of benefit in order for her to make her decision. I was surprised then, but having young children of my own now, I think I understand her choice better.

A particularly traumatic experience occurred while I was delivering bad news as an oncology fellow on the oncology inpatient consultation service. I explained to a patient and his family that although the surgeon was recommending chemotherapy to potentially reduce a tumor before surgery, the reality was that because of the degree of lymph node involvement of the gastric cancer, the intent of the chemotherapy was actually palliative. Understandably, the patient's daughter became upset. This information amounted to a paradigm shift in their understanding of the situation, and the daughter be-came verbally abusive, which eventually led me to tears. They were clearly not ready to hear this information, but I still struggle with whether or not it would have been acceptable for them to leave the institution with the wrong information. Equally difficult situations may arise when a patient's poor condition necessitates that a physi-cian deliver a poor prognosis before having a chance to develop a relationship, because the patient's decline may be imminent. In an-other case, a patient and her family left my care even after develop-ing a relationship with me because I attempted to discuss prognosis with them and they didn't want to hear it. Her husband pulled me aside and told me, "Her hope is the only thing keeping her from entering a severe depression."

Family members have asked me how much they or I should tell the patient. I tell them the truth and that is "I don't know." Where is that darn formula? I think most terminally ill cancer patients know that they will die sooner rather than later, and I think if it were me, I would not need to be told more than once. In her 2008 contribu-tion to the "The Art of Oncology: When the Tumor Is Not the Tar-get," Prudence Francis, who is a medical oncologist, wrote about her experience with a breast cancer patient who had asked her to be more optimistic about her prognosis: "This patient was made aware of her overall prognosis and the incurability of her disease . . . I never lied to my patient at any point about the potential benefits of therapy, but appropriately tempered my approach to avoid beating her over the head with poor prognosis talk at every juncture along the way. I believe that my patient had her eyes wide open, but pre-ferred to wear rose-colored glasses."[5]

Just recently, I had a similar experience with one of my colleagues' patients who was being enrolled in a clinical trial. As she had come to the trial "looking for a cure," I felt that it was my obligation to stress to her that this early-phase clinical trial, testing a new therapy, was not going to provide her a "cure." She reminded me that she had already beaten the odds, was a three-year survivor with metastatic pancreatic cancer, and stressed that she needed me to be on "her team" and "believe" that the therapy would work. She had been living with this diagnosis for three years and she knew the statistics all too well, but she needed me to participate in her optimistic framework. Being optimistic does not require one to be dishonest.

There is a selfish reason to disclose prognosis as early as possible, with frequent reinforcement. We wish to give patients and families time to come to grips with the reality that death is coming, and we hope that this will lead to the avoidance of heroic measures or unfruitful therapies in the early stages of dying. Unfortunately, despite our knowledge that metastatic pancreatic cancer portends a poor prognosis and a short survival, events leading to a patient's decline almost always still feel precipitous to the patient and the family. We frequently hear "I felt okay a few weeks ago and this took me by surprise." I fear that, even though Michael has had some time to contemplate these issues, a decline may still feel somewhat sudden to him and Beth, but I am glad that he has had the time to prepare his wishes.

FEELINGS ABOUT DEATH

Writing this book with Michael has been eye opening. He has never discussed with me his fears about dying, although he asked about the process of dying and what cancer patients actually die from. Despite dealing with dying patients on a regular basis, I do not feel equipped to guide them through the emotional and spiritual aspects of their illness. I acknowledge these shortcomings. For my own self-preservation and endurance in the field of oncology, I am grateful that I have a team to consult when I feel out of my element or feel that the patient needs more time than I might be able to provide. That team includes the oncology nurses, psychiatry liaison nurse, social workers, the pain and palliative care team, the hospice teams, and the pastoral care staff.

One thing I can do is listen, and that I try to do. Several of my patients have asked me what people with pancreatic cancer die from and what other symptoms will occur in their final weeks. I used to tell them about how some patients die from infection, others from blood clots, others from liver failure due to cancer infiltration, and still others from starvation due to bowel obstruction. I will still tell them about these processes if that is what I think they are really asking. But, in retrospect, and after reading Michael's perspective, I wonder if they are really asking, "How will I die"—not the physiology behind it, but if it will be a "good death." Will there be pain and will they suffer? I may take the opportunity to attempt to reassure them that we are partners and that I will be honest with them about when I think the treatment isn't worth the potential benefit, not only in regards to chemotherapy but also regarding supportive measures, such as artificial nutrition. I hope that I am able to allay some fears by reassuring patients that control of their anxiety and physical symptoms is of utmost importance to me and the medical staff in their remaining time. Aggressive pain management will be implemented to control pain and ensure a dignified death.

Michael's story also gives me a different insight into the tensions that I have seen between patients and their spouses. The interactions I've observed between spouses have vacillated between unending mutual support to a relationship that seemed more like parent and child. I think I would not have noticed this and similar behaviors in my patients if I had not read Michael's reflections on his increasing demands on Beth. His account is so powerful and honest that I think other patients and their caregivers may be able to gain some insight into some of their own conflicts.

These conflicts must also be viewed from the perspective of the caregiver. Caregivers are often at increased risk for depression and illness. More than half of caregivers are women. Coping with Michael's illness and his reaction to the illness has no doubt been a challenge for Beth. Members of the oncology team are available not only to the patients but to their family members as well. There are Internet resources as well, such as the Web sites Share the Care, Caring from a Distance, and PanCAN (Pancreatic Cancer Action

Network),[6] which has a section dedicated to caregivers. Caregiving takes a great deal of effort and selflessness and can often lead to burnout. Feelings of guilt, anger, and isolation are not uncommon. While advising caregivers to take care of themselves as well may seem intuitive, caregivers may need permission to or an order to take care of their own well-being before they feel comfortable doing so. They put the demands of the patient first, and it is often difficult for them to spend time and energy on themselves. Caregivers should try to find some time to focus on their own physical and mental health and to locate individuals or a support network with whom to commiserate.

7

Family and Friends

Writing about family is difficult for me. Writing about death focuses on how *I alone* am feeling. It is also talking about something that is still not quite real. Talking about family is talking about others, most of whom are close in some way. It brings up history that is both good and bad, and may be painful. Writing about these people probably will influence what happens in interactions among them and with me in the future.

In this chapter, as in other chapters, I describe personal situations. It is not that I enjoy revealing private aspects of my life, but I believe that the reader needs a concrete picture of the kinds of issues that arise when cancer strikes.

While there is heartache, and despair, when you receive a cancer diagnosis, and when you learn that you have only a short time more in this world, there is also a kind of opportunity. The chance to strengthen relationships within the family that have weakened over the years is one of the most valuable opportunities. This happened with me. Receiving the love and concern of family and friends is heartwarming. Being able to return it gives added meaning to your life.

THE SUPPORT OF FAMILY

There is nothing new about the idea that the support of family and friends is important after a diagnosis of cancer. Most people seem to have this support. It is often an extension of the love that existed before the diagnosis, and it may be intensified by the changed circumstances.

However, sad to say, not all family members and friends will step up to the plate to help the diagnosed person in the way he or she might wish. The disappointment can be hurtful when a family member's response is not as hoped for. Sometimes the patient disappoints family or friends during this final stage of life. This can be painful for them.

One of the cancer patients Beth and I both know has struggled with the response of her family, some of whom have remained more distant from her than she would like.[1] She has found support through her many friends, but it still hurts that those she expected the most from have not been closer and that they appear to consider her illness less important than mundane, everyday chores. We know that these relationships are not always black and white and that it takes understanding from both sides.

Small things, like a note from a colleague or a friend, mean a lot. Big things, like your kids wanting to come to see you, mean even more.

As I have said, I am not a religious man. One of my cousins, a rabbi with whom I have not been in touch since he was a teenager, wrote to tell me about Jewish tradition in a situation like mine. This touched me. I also know that my name is mentioned in churches and that friends all over the world say prayers for me. This also means a lot.

As I began to tell my family and friends of my diagnosis, first by e-mail and then by phone, I tried to be low-key, but people knew that pancreatic cancer is fatal and that the time horizon might be short.

My brother Stuart and sister-in-law Norma came from nearby Bethesda, Maryland, for a few hours. My sister Laurie flew in from

California. My son Motaki came for a quick visit, after Christmas, from North Carolina. It was exhausting, but I was happy to see each of them.

I wanted to tell friends what was happening, but I was often too weak to write. I asked Beth to take over after my first e-mails. She sent out long, detailed messages on how I was and what we were doing. She did not know many of the people to whom she was writing, which made the task difficult.

We also had a list of family and close friends to whom she wrote separately. To some who wished to come and see me, but were asked to wait a bit, it may have seemed that she was screening my contacts with the outside world. In fact, she was only carrying out my wishes. That was before we had heard of CaringBridge, a Web site[7] on which you can tell people what is going on without the need for individual e-mails. Of course, the message you post still has to be thought through.

The support I received in response to these communications was heartwarming. It *did* help. The power of e-mails was immense. I am used to communicating more by e-mail than by anything else, so this is especially true for me. It lifted my spirits. I could feel that people cared.

The first reactions to my diagnosis were deep concern and sympathy. Three of my four kids (they will always be kids, even though they are in their thirties and forties) live overseas. They wanted to come right away. However, I did not want that until we knew more about what was going to happen.

We were traveling to Baltimore for my chemotherapy two weeks out of every three. At first, we stayed several nights each week in Baltimore as we tried to gauge my reaction to the chemotherapy. Because we are not close to an emergency medical facility that we had confidence in (rightly or wrongly) where we live in West Virginia, we felt more comfortable with this routine. Many things were going on at the same time that first December and January. I believed that having more visitors would be too difficult.

I admit I was of two minds on this. I wanted my children to come because I loved them and I knew my diagnosis was grave and had been a shock to them, and that my time might be very limited. At the same time, I was not sure I wanted anyone to come. Much of the time I wanted to be alone, and I wanted to be able to set the pace of visiting. I was single-minded about getting my affairs in order. And I *was* exhausted most of the time.

I managed to persuade my children not to come until we knew more about what the course of events would be. They understood but were worried. Being far away probably made them feel helpless.

Often, the caregiver must be the one to set limits on visiting and communications. In my case, Beth stepped forward, for which I was thankful.

Close relatives are easily hurt when they think they are not wanted. The reason for delaying seeing some people is not that you do not love them. It is only that visits can be overwhelming, for different reasons at various stages of having cancer.

I was unprepared for the family problems created by my diagnosis: the questions of whom to call and who should be allowed to visit. I had not thought about the issues, had not expected them, and was not prepared for them. None of us was. No one ever is, really.

After diagnosis I began chemotherapy very quickly. I felt awful and was weak. I did not want to face up to my emotions or to worry about anyone coming to see me. I was quickly exhausted; thirty minutes of being with anyone except Beth was my maximum. I was not an invalid, although during the first few weeks of chemo I did spend a lot of time in my pajamas. Having company required us to prepare, no matter how thoughtful everyone tried to be, and neither Beth nor I was up to a stream of visitors.

I was not yet on my deathbed, but I thought that having visitors would be awkward. Actually, the problem was more in the way I imagined it might be rather than the reality. I worried that we might look at each other, not knowing quite what to say. Being more solitary seemed more appealing to me. That was the way I had always been. Each person must be true to himself or herself. There is no right way.

I was ill then, but when I was able to withstand the first dose of chemo, Dr. Le increased it. This dosing decision had significant benefits, but the price was feeling just plain awful. Still, I am of the school that believes that if there is no suffering there is probably not that much happening inside. I felt better feeling bad than I would have if I had sailed through the chemo.

MEDICAL UPDATE

In mid-February 2008, I had the first scan since my diagnosis. We saw Dr. Le that same day. She had very good news. The chemo was working. The tumors were smaller. The CA19-9 had also gone down dramatically.

Beth remembers when Dr. Le told us this. We sat in silence. She had to say "Guys, this is good news" before we began to smile. I had not dared to think this might happen. It was unexpected. We had not wanted to hope too much, for fear of being disappointed.

CA19-9 results have become a very important part of my life. CA19-9 is a substance in the blood that indicates pancreatic cancer tumor activity. The higher the CA19-9 number, the more active the cancer. The test for CA19-9 is a very useful test, but it is not reliable for all people who have this cancer (and, unfortunately, it is not a test that can be used for early screening for the disease). Over time, we learned, to my relief, that for me the test is a reliable indicator of what my tumors are doing or not doing. It has always correlated closely with what my scans show about the tumors. As the tumors shrink, so does my CA19-9 number.

In early December 2007, my CA19-9 reading had been in the 5000 range. A normal reading is between 0 and 36. By the end of January, after being treated for a little more than a month, it had dropped more than 60 percent, to about 1700. It continued to drop. At the same time, the first postdiagnostic scan, in February, confirmed that the tumors were smaller.

I knew these results meant a reprieve, of sorts. I was not going to die immediately. I also knew this could change at any moment. Some things I had read emphasized the ability of cancer cells to mutate, in which case treatments that have been effective become less so.

So, while we were relieved about the immediate impact of the GTX treatments, we remained very cautious. There was no change in my diagnosis. The cancer had metastasized. It would always be stage IV pancreatic cancer.

In response to worsening side effects, Dr. Le began to reduce the high doses of the chemotherapy drugs. She also began to cut back on the amount of steroid medication I was being given on the days before and after chemo. I began to feel a little better. I knew that death was inevitable, but maybe it would not happen as quickly as I had thought.

A number of things loomed large at this point. We write about them here in consecutive chapters, but the truth is that everything was going on more or less simultaneously: tasks and goals, thinking about death, worrying about family, trying to make it through each day, the exhausting routine of going back and forth for treatment, acquiring strange new medical knowledge, and trying to hold things together at home were just a few of the things going on at the same time in my life and brain and spirit. In spite of the improvement in my CA19-9, I still had an overwhelming sense of melancholy and lassitude. I was immensely sad. Indeed, who would not be, in this situation?

My mood improved when Dr. Le prescribed an antidepressant, bupropion. This medication course had a bumpy start. I misunderstood the number of pills to be taken. Instead of taking one pill every twelve hours, I took two pills when I got up in the morning. This went on for a couple of weeks. By midmorning I became ravenously hungry. I could not get enough to eat. This was good for regaining lost weight, since I was very thin at this point, as are many cancer patients. But that dose of the medication also put me on edge.

Somehow, this mistake came to light, and so one problem, at least, was solved. Everything improved after that.

While I was getting my chemotherapy treatments, Beth was able to talk to one of the social workers at the hospital, and this was a support for her. I am sure we do not take full advantage of all that the hospital has on offer, but we know we can ask for more support if we need it.

At home, I realized that I needed to get up and out more than I had been, and to start doing a few things around the house. The diagnosis and the need for twenty-four-hour care, followed by my behaving like I was very dependent when I did not really need to be, had been hard on Beth. I began to think about what I should be doing over the next few months. I began to think more about my kids.

FAMILY HISTORY AND FAMILY ISSUES

Here, I need to say a little more about my own background. In the late 1960s, I had been a Peace Corps volunteer in Botswana, in southern Africa. I got married there. My wife already had three children, all boys, whom I adopted. We subsequently had one child together, four sons in all—Motaki, Thoko, Thapelo, and Leungo.

Eventually we came to the United States. My career took me all over the world, although we lived mainly in Africa. The kids grew up and struck out on their own. Each is successful in his own way and in his own chosen field. Motaki, the oldest, is a pharmacist in North Carolina. Thoko is an economic development consultant in Botswana. Thapelo, also in Botswana, is a telecommunications expert and has been the CEO of two large companies there. Leungo, the youngest, is a chef in New Zealand. I love and am proud of all of them.

My first wife and I separated in 1992 and divorced in 1997. Beth and I met in 2002, married in 2003, and moved that same year to West Virginia. Beth is a retired schoolteacher. For part of her career, she taught students who were too sick to attend public school. Some of these students had cancer. She had learned a lot about the needs of cancer patients and about what to do and not do when one is around them.

At the time of my diagnosis, my first wife lived not far away, in Washington, D.C. We had not been in touch since my remarriage. Both Beth and I thought she should be included in communications about my health, but there were tensions almost immediately. In the midst of all our other worries, I found myself trying to mediate misunderstandings.

I had learned as a volunteer mediator in the Small Claims Court of the District of Columbia that one should never mediate a case in which one is personally involved. Nevertheless, I tried to do this. All the difficulties that might have been expected arose. I doubt if anyone was happy with how that attempt at communication worked out.

I had read somewhere that marriages often suffer during the period right after a cancer diagnosis, and this was true of Beth and me. The strains were enormous. My anger, masked though it might have been, added further stress, as did my sense of entitlement.

Beth was responsible for my survival during this period. The position of the caregiver who is also obliged by circumstance to deal with the family of the patient is always a delicate one. I felt that everyone was doing the best that could be expected under difficult circumstances, but not everyone agreed. Beth soldiered on as my sole caregiver and took good care of me at an especially sensitive time.

My own family, the Lippes, have never been the kind of family who keep up with each other by regular phone calls. We seem to be more comfortable living our own lives and assuming that everything is okay with everyone else. At least, that is how I am, or was, and I assumed that my brother and sister were the same. This is how we had acted with one another, even though it might not have been how we acted with others. We each have, as does everyone, baggage we carry from childhood.

Long periods, sometimes years, passed when the Lippes did not see one another. We lived in different parts of the world and it was not easy to keep in touch. In our family, it did not seem wrong if we did not make a great effort. I remember a time in 1991 toward the end of my mother's life when she was ill with leukemia. She had taken a particularly bad turn, nearly dying. We lived in Kenya at the time. Instead of picking up the phone and calling, my father wrote me a letter. Because of the Gulf War, mail was delayed and the letter didn't arrive until six weeks later. I phoned immediately. I learned that my mother had survived, but she then passed away before my next visit to their home in Florida, only several months later. I regret terribly that we had not kept in closer touch.

This was my model for how things were done in situations like the one I now faced. It is not that we do not love each other. We do. We just do not communicate as I imagine most other families do. I might be wrong; maybe our way is not so unusual. In any event, I always wanted something different. I did not know how to get it and I certainly did not work at it.

This was what I knew, and without thinking about it, I had probably continued this model with my own kids. I loved them and was sure they loved me, but communicating with each other, by phone or letters was another matter. Although I talked with them more than my parents had talked with me, it was still probably not enough.

My way of connecting with family as an adult has been to bond with the families of my wives or the person I was with.

Beth comes from a very different kind of family, a southern family from a culture far different from mine. Beth is very close to her mother and sister. Today, as her mother ages, she telephones her almost every day. They chat about all the things going on in their daily lives, what each is having for supper, what the weather is, what has happened to the dogs next door—the small events of everyday life. Consequently, they know pretty much what is happening in each other's lives on a daily and weekly basis. The Lippes do not.

I love to listen to these conversations. They are a part of family living that I never knew. During the conversations, if there is something important that has to be discussed, it is. My health became the most important concern for Beth's family. I enjoy being a part of this kind of family. At the same time, I do not want to idealize them unrealistically. There are disagreements and problems, but a basic tolerance and concern for the well-being of each family member prevails.

When I found out that I had cancer, I had to decide how to tell my family. There really was not that much to decide. E-mail seemed the only way. I was afraid of shocking them with a phone call and afraid I might not know what to say nor how to say it over the phone. Facing emotion head-on was difficult. I e-mailed everyone. And then I followed up with my kids by phone.

Beth immediately picked up the phone and called her family. I doubt if it ever occurred to her to do anything else. Even if it had been she who had been diagnosed, this is what she would have done. Of course, one phone call was all it took to start the ball rolling, as one person called another and another.

There are as many ways of telling families about a cancer diagnosis as there are families. There may be no best way. I bring up my family and Beth's family only as two examples among many, so that it is clear there are great differences among families. The important thing is that everyone who needs to know is told.

However, not everyone needs to know. One acquaintance of mine kept her cancer a secret from her aging and ill mother, because she felt her mother's knowing might have dire consequences.

I mentioned briefly in Chapter 5 an example—an older lady writing a long letter—of something helpful that can be done, like drafting your will, immediately after diagnosis. It is also an example of one way to tell friends and family of your diagnosis. That lady had breast cancer and had had a mastectomy. She was in her eighties and did not expect to survive very long. Nevertheless, years passed before her death. Finally, she began to have pains in her back. She was told that the cancer had come back. It had metastasized to her bones. There was nothing to do, they said. She was of an advanced age, too old to treat.

She went home and thought about how to tell everyone she knew. She decided the best way was to write a letter to everyone. This was in the early 1990s. I did not see the letter, but here is how my friend who told me the story described the situation:

> She went into the doctor's office and I guess this was when they did a biopsy, and he said that the cancer had come back . . . He didn't give her a timeline but said that without treatment it was going to be terminal . . . She came home and she got me to help her write a letter. And the letter was to go out to this whole list of her friends and her family and friends of mine and everybody she knew. And she told them that her cancer had come back and she was dying and not to feel bad for her because she had had a wonderful life . . . She didn't want anybody to feel they hadn't done enough for her or that they hadn't seen her enough . . . the gift to her was that they had been in her life and she had known them, and had appreciated them.[3]

This was a moving farewell. As one can imagine, there was an outpouring of love in response to her letter. One person brought her a book that had just come out, *Cold Mountain*, set in her native North Carolina. Another person called up the local Baskin-Robbins and had her sent ten pints of ice cream. There were many wonderful testimonials of support.

That is not the end of the story. Perhaps this outpouring helped the old lady (whose hair was always dyed red). She lived on for many years, a second time, enjoying these memories. In fact, after several years she began to wonder whether she ought to send out another letter!

This outpouring was like one I experienced, in some ways. In writing this book, I asked my kids to try to recall their reactions upon hearing of my diagnosis. Leungo wrote from New Zealand, "It was a normal morning in Wanaka. I had dropped Clover to school and Lisa to work and I was at home with Xion. The phone rang and it was Michael [he calls me by my first name]. From what I can remember, he didn't waste time in breaking the news . . . The memory has faded, but the emotion I felt after that was overwhelming. The main thing was I wanted to go and be of aid in any way possible. I remember after getting off the phone, I didn't even call Lisa, I kinda just sat there with Xi and shook my head. It was not until I picked her up that I told her about the call. Lisa had to drive home, I was pretty broken."[4]

Thapelo, who lives in Botswana, wrote, "I remember my father's words as if he's saying them right now; however I couldn't tell you what day of the year it was or the time of day. The message came like any other from my father, well measured, calm and ironically nurturing; the crux, he'd been diagnosed with stage IV pancreatic cancer. If ever all intricacies of the mind were ablaze with activity beyond my control, it was then . . . While all hell was literally breaking loose in my head, I maintained the type of calm my father had endowed me with. I listened intently, thankful that we were talking over the phone as I knew I would not have been as strong as I was in person."[5]

The day I made those calls, I could feel their love and this helped me. But there were also issues to surmount. Although my kids wanted to come see me, and this meant a lot to me, Beth and I were not ready. We were too busy trying to stabilize my health. We were in Baltimore two weeks out of three for several days at a time and we were exhausted from the chemo and the traveling. We had moved houses and were trying to settle in to the new place.

I said no, this was not the right time to come. I believed there would be time for them to come, later on. This disappointed my kids, I am sure, but my belief proved accurate, as my February scan showed I was stabilizing. For me, however, just knowing that people wanted to come was almost as supportive as their coming.

I guess there is no easy way to make sure that everyone understands what the situation is, and everyone you tell will react differently. Many times, it seems to us, this reaction depends more on how the *others* feel than how the person who is sick feels. The fact is, there are going to be issues and friction. What is needed, when telling people about your diagnosis, is to be clear and honest. Try to make everyone understand your needs.

This is easy to say, but not so easy to do.

My brother began to call once or twice a week. This changed our relationship. In the beginning, we hardly knew what to say to each other, it had been so long since we had talked in any real way, but gradually the conversations became more personal. They never matched Beth's easygoing conversations with her mother and sister, but they were a positive change that I appreciated and looked forward to. Even though my health has improved, we have continued to talk.

My sister wanted to call and talk as often as I would allow. Again, this was important to me. My Uncle Dan and Aunt Naomi came to visit from Chicago for several days, after the chemo began to work. They helped Beth by taking me to have my blood drawn, which meant one less thing Beth had to do. Leungo and his family came in April of 2008. Thapelo came in July. He took me to Baltimore for chemotherapy. It turned out to be one of the few times I was unable to have a treatment because my white cell blood counts were too low, but at least it gave him a first-hand look at some of the things that happen during therapy. These visits, although sometimes stressful, helped me.

Beth and her mother talked every day about how I was doing. I listened to these conversations and they made me stronger. They nourished me. I would ask every day if Beth had talked to her mother yet.

There was something about these conversations that Beth noticed. She would ask me if I wanted to talk, too. I didn't. Just hearing her side of the conversation was all I needed. I guess I was still one step removed from this kind of familiarity with family. I was still an outsider, and more comfortable in that position.

Beth's sister, Nan, did an enormous amount of research for us on the Internet about pancreatic cancer, research that Beth did not have the time or sometimes, she said, the courage, to do. Sometimes one finds out more than is needed, and we found it helpful for someone else to sift through and get to the core of the information we were interested in.

Nan's husband Tom, our brother-in-law, was kind and caring, and encouraging as well. When we arrived in North Carolina that first January after my diagnosis, and on other subsequent visits, he ran errands for us, no matter how trivial. For Beth, this was responsibility shared and she was very appreciative of this help.

The support from friends and colleagues was almost all done by e-mail, and it was comforting to realize that my life had been worth something to so many people.

I was prayed for in almost every religion and in many different languages, since I had known people from many different countries and backgrounds through my work.

I began to think about regrets I had, and harms I had caused, and to wonder whether there was anything I might do about them before it was too late. I was somewhat familiar with Al-Anon and with the twelve-step program, which includes reaching out to those you may have harmed. As in many other things, I am afraid, I fall short in actually doing this. However, I made a beginning.

During all this, chemo continued to be rough, and by March 2008 Beth was overwhelmed and exhausted. Seeing my kids meant so much to me, but the timing turned out to be problematic. Beth had devoted all her time and energy to my care for three months and needed to catch up with her own pressing matters, which included medical issues and other things she had been forced to neglect. I, however, deferred to my kids' schedules. Beth felt she was pushed to the edge, and that having responsibilities for others, even her stepchildren, was more than she could handle.

This is an example of how worn down even a dedicated caregiver can become and how important it is to reach compromises on issues like visitors. The other thing that became clear was the need to reach an agreement with visitors on who would be responsible for what during the visit.

My response was to assume that we could, and would, manage. This was selfish. All I can say now, as I look back, is that I thought I did not have much time left, and I was ready to have my children come; I wanted them as near to me as possible. When you are very ill, your own needs and desires occupy more of your time and energy, and thinking about the needs of others is harder than when you are healthy.

There was something else I wanted which I had been thinking about for some time. It became an obsession after my scan in February 2008 showed an improvement. This desire had taken hold as I made progress with my will and as my health had gradually improved.

I wanted a new car. Actually, I had wanted one for several years. We had two cars already. Beth did not want me to drive at all because I was still wobbly and the automobile insurance is in her name. She was right, but I wanted what I wanted. I began to look at leasing a car.

Eventually, I got a little VW beetle convertible, on a thirty-month lease. I told everyone that I was determined to live to the end of the lease, in order not to lose money on it. It became a goal.

However, because Beth had opposed the idea, I decided to do it on my own, without telling her. I guess I expected that she would accept a fait accompli, or maybe I wanted this so much that I did not care about her objections. There it was, sitting in the driveway when she returned, unsuspecting, from a trip to Chicago for her own medical care.

She realized immediately that I had not told the truth when she called me from the headache clinic in Chicago to find out how I was feeling. Leungo and his family had come to visit at the time, in early April. He was unaware of the intrigue. We had driven up to get the new car and to go to a mall. When I took her call on my cell phone, I told her we were at the mall, when in fact I was signing the lease for the car at that very moment. She was very angry, and rightly so. Moreover, she made sure I knew it then and for the next two years. She refused to ride in the car . . . ever.

Nevertheless, driving this car up and down our road, with the top down, made *me* immensely happy. It was wonderful therapy. I tell this story, embarrassing though it is, to illustrate the kinds of ins and outs that persons on this journey will encounter. I was wrong to lie, and yet not wrong to have leased the car. Beth was right, and yet not right. There will be these ambiguities.

These were not happy times at home, and I didn't make them easier. My feelings of entitlement, my hidden anger at Beth, grappling with family issues, and the relentless chemo schedule, all crowded into front and center. They comprised my daily existence.

LESSONS ABOUT VISITORS

One issue that Beth has raised and that I agree with, though I understood it too late, is that an overburdened caregiver needs support, not the added burden of catering to even more people. My time horizon was short, but that is not an excuse that trumps all other considerations. A more balanced approach would have been better.

We did not try this approach, but looking back, I realize it is a commonsense one. Let visitors know before they arrive that they will need to help out. Decide with them in advance what supporting roles they will assume.

Even for visitors who come for only part of the day, following a few house rules will make the visit more enjoyable, and less frustrating, for everyone. Timeliness is the most important of these. Arriving on time and leaving on time, especially when the patient is very weak, can make all the difference in the world. At times, I would be exhausted just by sitting. If Beth joined in the visit, she would be obliged to delay or omit tasks that needed to be done that day.

THE SUPPORT OF FRIENDS

The trips to Baltimore seemed endless, but there was one thing about them that we looked forward to. We stayed at the Marriott Waterfront hotel, at a special Hopkins rate, and this allowed for a bit of rest Beth could not otherwise get. Neither of us felt like rushing back home after the chemotherapy treatments. Beth had cataracts at the time and could not drive at night, and I cannot drive after treatments. We thought about renting an apartment in Baltimore, but that seemed impossible given our responsibilities in West Virginia. This turned out to be one of those little decisions that pays off handsomely in the end. Looking back, the hotel stays were the best thing we could have done for ourselves at that time. Being able to have relatively stress-free chemo sessions, rather than rushing in and out of town, seemed to us to be the right choice, and even now we spend the night before chemo at the hotel.

I remember thinking how hard it must be for some of the people who would drive several hours for their chemo and then have to go back that same day in the afternoon. I was exhausted and so was Beth. Reflecting on this, I wonder if the hotel stays are not part of the reason my body has accepted treatment so readily.

For us, the hotel became our friend. Of course, it is the people in the hotel, the staff collectively, who have made it seem this way. Although it was a chore to go to Baltimore, when we arrived at the Waterfront we felt a relaxation, even peacefulness, not always possible at home.

Our welcome was always warm. We felt it was real. Everyone knew my story. Andy the doorman, with whom Beth found a common interest in gardening, brought us flowers from his garden. On one stay, we even went to his house, and met his wife, who picked flowers for us to take to North Carolina for Beth's mother. Reggie, another doorman, was always cheerful and helpful. He helped Beth squeeze everything into the back of our car and arrange the dog pillows for me to ride on during that first trip to North Carolina, so I could have my little perch in the back seat. Kate Jenkins, Nick, Guss, Trang, Sinead, the Rumanian girls, and all the others at the desk gave us an upgraded room on almost every stay. Once, knowing that it was our anniversary, they sent flowers to us, along with chocolate covered strawberries and sparkling cider! Their kindnesses are too numerous to list. Concerned porters help us with our luggage. The huge flower displays in the lobby are always soothing. Valets take our car and always ask how "Mr. Mike" is doing. Fulgence, from the Ivory Coast, brings us a small fridge many weeks. I speak French with him in that warm West African way that I got used to when I lived there years ago. Marlene Marriott from Jamaica is the welcoming presence in the concierge lounge. She lavishes us with kindness and warmth, and keeps in touch when our paths do not cross for some reason. She is also someone we can confide in, and have.

Everyone knows our story and everyone is on our side. All of this is great for my morale and, just as important, for Beth's morale.

Another side of the support we have received concerns friends in West Virginia. We moved here in 2003. Even though it was only 60 miles from where we had lived, it is a very different world. In response to my illness, we have been shown a warmth that is hard to imagine receiving had we remained in the big city.

I think about the people who are so kind to us. One example is typical. I remember one evening remarking to Beth about the wonderful flounder we had just had for dinner. I knew it had come from Les and Ali. Les and Ali have their fish stand in the parking area of a gas station outside Harper's Ferry. They set up every weekend from roughly Easter to late fall, bringing seafood from the coast. Beth told me that when she had asked Les how much she owed for the fish and for the sunflowers from his parents' farm nearby, he had named a figure that she knew was too low. She asked again, saying that the amount didn't add up. Les said he knew, but he also knew where it was going. And that was that. I do not know if we enjoyed the weekly fish and sunflowers more because of this act of generosity, but we certainly looked forward to both every week.

This is the sort of thing that sustains Beth and me.

Over the years we have lived in Shepherdstown, we have tried to get as much of our food as possible from local producers. It tastes better, is healthier, and helps support the local economy. This means going to the farmers' market every Sunday we are home. After five years, we know many of the farmers who come every week. Their concern for me and their sympathy for Beth are especially comforting. She feels they are a part of our caring team.

We have a routine in the market and in other nearby places that makes for a certain rhythm in our small town life. We go to Jimi for tomatoes, Mike and Krissy for vegetables (we visited their farm once in Maryland with my granddaughter from Philadelphia), Bill for meat and vegetables, Erland for salad and cucumbers, Amy for cookies and peanuts, and Megan for flowers (she had provided flowers for our wedding in 2003). When the local town council tried to impose new regulations on the market, we went to the town meeting and I spoke up in favor of the farmers. They did not forget this act of solidarity.

We also travel across the Potomac River to Washington County, Maryland, to Burkeholders' Bakery and then on to Mr. Lanham's for the best bicolored corn around. As with the farmers' market, people came to know our story and were caring and supportive. Our local post office, where we go almost every day and see Willy, Louise, Sandy, and Kandy, and many others from the town, is also a constant source of support. Our small local library, where Hali Taylor is the director and where Brenda Burlin worked, before her recent death after many years of living with breast cancer, has played an important role in our life. And then there are Butch and Linda Homsher, our friends from Marlowe, who have served as our guides to life in West Virginia.

My purpose is not to try to name all the people in town who are nice to us. It is to show that this is the kind of support that is heart-warming and can be life preserving. It is the kind of support that should be sought if not volunteered but which frequently comes unsolicited when you need it most.

The blood marker CA19-9 passed into the normal range in May and my scans showed that the tumors were continuing to shrink. Physically, I had come through the initial months.

Emotionally, I still needed to come to grips with many issues. I had drawn closer to family and friends, and this was good, but I still needed to find my way out of the unhappiness that persisted during most of 2008, much of it self-inflicted.

8

Managing the Symptoms of Advanced Cancer

There were early signs that Michael was responding to therapy. His CA19-9 had declined by 15 percent after one cycle of therapy (two weekly infusions followed by a week without) and by 60 percent after two cycles of therapy. In addition, his pain was decreasing. I was confident that his CT scans, which were scheduled after his third cycle, would show that the tumor status was at the very least stable. Although I have been fooled by tumor marker declines in the past, Michael's results were as I expected. Both his liver and pancreatic tumors showed a slight decrease in size since the previous examination. I would also have been pleased with the scans if they had only showed stable tumor sizes, as I believe that lack of tumor growth translates to improved outcomes for patients. I started him at a slightly lower dose of Xeloda than generally prescribed, to make sure he could tolerate it, and then I increased his dose to the full amount. Over time we had to lower the doses of all the drugs because of bone marrow toxicity.

As Michael was slugging through the treatments, I was able to get to know him and Beth. With each dose reduction, I could sense a concern from him that a reduction in dose would mean a reduction in disease-fighting efficacy. This thoughtful questioning gave me insight into Michael's feelings. The amount of side effects he was experiencing was acceptable to him as long as things seemed to be working.

At every point in the care of an oncology patient, there are many important issues to address other than antitumor therapies. Attention to attempts to control the cancer should not detract from the very important aspects of the supportive care required by most patients with cancer. Supportive and palliative care begin with the initial diagnosis and continue throughout treatment, during periods of disease progression and during periods of remission. Some of the issues addressed by supportive care are common to many cancer types, for example, depression and/or anxiety, management of pain, nutrition, management of fluid collections in the abdominal and chest cavities, and introduction to hospice care. There are also some issues that are more specific to pancreatic cancer, such as pancreatic insufficiency and management of biliary obstruction. In addition, most patients with pancreatic cancer have underlying medical conditions, like hypertension and diabetes, which require monitoring and adjustments of medications during therapy.

Michael has already experienced some of these commonly encountered issues. Fortunately, he is not destined to experience all of the symptoms discussed below, but a vast majority of cancer patients will develop some of these problems at some point in their journey.

DEPRESSION AND ANXIETY

For many years, we have known that there is a link between pancreatic cancer and depression. From 30 percent to 70 percent of pancreatic cancer patients also experience depression. The association is sufficiently strong that physicians taking care of patients with pancreatic cancer should look for depression in their patients. In fact, some studies suggest that symptoms of depression and anxiety can predate the diagnosis of pancreatic cancer by months or even years.[1] While clinical depression is seen in people with various types of cancer, it is significantly more common in those with pancreatic cancer. While the physical mechanisms of this depression are not completely worked out, data suggest that the higher levels of cytokines, or proteins, in the blood of pancreatic cancer patients play a potential role in the development of depression in these people.

Depression can have a significant impact on a patient's quality of life. It can influence the coping mechanisms needed to deal with mood, anxiety, and pain, and it also has an impact on appetite and energy levels. Depression can present a variety of symptoms, including depressed mood, anxiety, and irritability. Patients can have insomnia (difficulty sleeping), hypersomnia (excess sleeping), loss of interest in usual activities, decreased appetite, weight loss, and fatigue. It is sometimes difficult to tease out when these symptoms are due to depression and when to cancer progression, but in truth, there is little harm done in trying to treat depression, regardless of its origin.

In treating depression, the counseling provided by social workers, psychotherapists, and palliative care teams is invaluable, but antidepressant medications are an additional option for patients. However, physicians do need to be mindful of the potential side effects of these medications, especially considering that the patient may already be struggling with negative side effects of chemotherapy. Because we do not have large studies to rely on to help choose the best antidepressants for patients with pancreatic cancer, the drug selection may come down to what the oncologist is familiar with in terms of prior experience and known toxicity profiles. Whether or not a patient is experiencing insomnia, has decreased appetite, or has a cardiac disease history may play into the treatment choice. Other considerations may include renal (kidney) or hepatic (liver) dysfunction. I try to use a drug that is covered by the patient's insurance and

I typically use one of the newer classes of antidepressants that act to regulate neurotransmitters. Neurotransmitters are chemicals released in the brain.

Most antidepressants take weeks or months to work, so dosing decisions need to be made with that in mind. I chose bupropion for Michael because I had come across a couple of small studies that suggested that it could help with cancer-related fatigue, which he was experiencing.[2]

Treating depressive symptoms can have many benefits. While basing decisions on anecdotes may not be scientific, I have had patients tell me, as Michael did, that their mood improved and they also became less argumentative with their spouses after starting antidepressant therapy. There are also patients who seem to eat a little better after being started on an antidepressant. I recently prescribed an antidepressant for a gentleman with pancreatic cancer who adamantly denied being depressed but who now, for the first time in many months, has an appetite. Of course, this does not mean I was right about his depressed mood, but at the very least, the medication did provide some appetite stimulation. There are others whose pain is better controlled when antidepressants are used as an adjunct to pain medications. Some medications, such as steroids, may exacerbate symptoms of depression, anxiety, or insomnia. Steroids are often given with antitumor therapies to decrease the risk of side effects from certain chemotherapeutic agents or to stimulate appetite. Eliminating or lowering doses of steroids may be necessary to prevent depressive symptoms.

The control of pain is intimately connected to depression. As you can imagine, uncontrolled pain can lead to anxiety, depression, and difficulty in coping.

CANCER PAIN

Pain is one of the most common symptoms of pancreatic cancer, and increases in pain cause a great deal of anxiety for patients and their caregivers. Pain management with opioid pain medications was discussed in Chapter 4. It is extremely important to adequately treat cancer pain, as it is one of the most distressing symptoms for patients. In addition to carefully adjusting opioid medications as previously described, the physician may try adjunct medications such as antidepressants, nonsteroidal anti-inflammatory drugs such as naproxen (Aleve), and antiseizure medicines such as gabapentin (Neurontin). The antiseizure medications are more likely to have an effect on nerve-based pain. I have had variable success with combinations of these adjunct medications, depending upon the individual patient. A short course of radiation may be delivered to a tumor to slow its growth and reduce pain, if the tumor is thought to be the culprit causing intense pain. An example of this would be a tumor that has metastasized to a bone and is causing pain there.

For patients with pancreatic cancer, physicians may consider a "pain block," which is also referred to as a celiac plexus or splanchnic nerve block with neurolysis. Early in my training, I was somewhat skeptical of these blocks, as I had a run of patients who did not seem to benefit from the intervention. All it took for me to reconsider was a handful of patients for whom a pain block provided significant relief from abdominal or back pain that had lasted for months. The procedure involves injection of alcohol or phenol into the nerves that supply the pancreas and surrounding areas. While there are some small risks in the procedure, I have not found the incidence of these risks to be sufficiently high to be of concern I think the most important risk is that it might not work, leaving the patient in as much pain but possibly more frustrated and discouraged. The medical risks include temporary low blood pressure, infection, and severe but short-term postprocedural pain. These blocks can be performed percutaneously (through the skin), intraoperatively (in the operating room), or endoscopically (using a scope introduced through the mouth and into the stomach).

In a study of 137 patients, those who had an intraoperative alcohol celiac plexus neurolysis experienced lower mean pain scores at two, four, and six months after pancreatic cancer surgery as compared to those who received only a salt water injection (or placebo).[3] A recent review in the *Journal of Clinical Gastroenterology* reported that endoscopic ultrasound-guided celiac plexus neurolysis was 72.5 percent effective in managing pain due to pancreatic cancer.[4] I believe this is a reasonable option for those who have developed tolerance to opioid analgesics and for those who cannot tolerate the side effects of opioids, such as fatigue, confusion, itching, urinary retention, and constipation. Typically, these blocks do not eliminate the need for opioids altogether, but they usually provide at least partial pain relief for a period of weeks to months.

BLOOD CLOTS

Pancreatic cancer is one of the cancers most commonly associated with blood clots. A pulmonary embolism or embolus (PE) is a blood clot in the lung, and a deep vein thrombosis (DVT) typically occurs in one of the large vessels in the legs. In some cases, a blood clot may be the first sign of pancreatic cancer.

Symptoms of pulmonary embolism include shortness of breath, chest pain, and cough. The shortness of breath often comes on suddenly and is present both at rest and with movement. The chest pain is often worse with a deep breath or cough. And the cough may be dry or bloody. With frequent CT scan imaging, more patients are being diagnosed with pulmonary emboli even before they show symptoms. Pulmonary emboli are most frequently diagnosed by CT scans using a special PE-specific protocol, but they can also be diagnosed by a nuclear medicine test called a ventilation/perfusion (V/Q) scan. This latter scan is particularly helpful in patients who cannot take the contrast dye required for the CT scan.

Symptoms of a DVT include swelling of the leg that may be accompanied by pain or redness in the leg. They are typically diagnosed by an ultrasound instrument called a Doppler. Deep vein thromboses can lead to pulmonary emboli, which can be life threatening.

The treatment for blood clots is anticoagulation or thinning of the blood. The anticoagulant is given to prevent further clot formation while the body's natural mechanisms dissolve the clot. Anti-coagulant treatment for pancreatic cancer patients may need to be lifelong, because the treatment should continue until the risk factors are no longer present.

The most commonly used anticoagulants are the warfarins and the heparins. Anticoagulation can come in pill form (warfarin, or Coumadin) or injection form (heparin or low-molecular-weight heparin). Warfarin does not work immediately and its effects have to be monitored periodically with a blood test, the INR, to guide dose adjustments. It should initially be administered with intravenous heparin or subcutaneous low-molecular-weight heparin (LMWH), as these work immediately. Common LMWHs include Lovenox and Fragmin. The benefit of LMWH is that, in stable patients, it can be administered on an outpatient basis because it is injected subcutaneously (just underneath the skin) and does not need to be monitored by an APTT test, which is needed to monitor intravenous heparin.

For patients who can accept daily injections of LMWH, the injections may be used instead of warfarin for longer term, maintenance treatment. Some studies have shown that in comparison to oral anticoagulants, LMWHs decrease the recurrence rates of clots without increasing the risk of bleeding.[5] However, LMWH is not always covered by insurance, because it is expensive, and the data regarding the survival benefit in patients with metastatic cancer is sparse.

Vena cava filters are sometimes used if patients cannot take blood thinners or they develop clots despite being on blood thinners. They are tiny umbrella-shaped filters placed in the inferior vena cava, a large blood vessel leading from the lower extremities, that prevent blood clots from moving from the leg veins to the lungs. However, a filter does not prevent the formation of more clots.

BILIARY OBSTRUCTION

Bile is a substance produced in the liver and transmitted through the biliary ducts into the intestines. It helps process fats, among other functions. Biliary obstruction from pancreatic cancer typically occurs when a tumor in the head of the pancreas blocks the common bile duct. This results in a back-up of bilirubin into the bloodstream, causing jaundice, or yellowing of the skin, and darkening of the urine as bilirubin is excreted into the urinary system. Because bile normally enters the stool, the lack of bile in the stool (acholic stools) can result in pale-colored stools. Blockage of a system that normally drains into the bowel can cause cholangitis, or infection of the biliary tree (the bile-draining ducts in the liver), which can be life threatening.

When biliary obstruction occurs, the blockage is usually reopened by inserting into the duct a stent or a biliary tube, devices that hold open the narrowed passageway, so that the bile can drain into the bowel. Biliary tubes are placed transcutaneously (through the skin), transhepatically (through the liver) by an interventional radiologist who uses sophisticated imaging to insert the drainage line through the skin and into the main draining bile duct. The tube typically empties into a plastic pouch that is placed on the outside of the skin. Once adequate drainage is achieved, the tube can be "internalized," which means that the end on the outside of the body is "capped" so that the bile will drain into the bowel instead. Biliary stents can also be used to reverse biliary obstruction. These devices expand to hold open the passageway and can be placed one of two ways, either endoscopically or transcutaneously. The first method is done by a trained gastroenterologist, who puts an endoscope, a long, thin tube, through the patient's mouth, down into the stomach, and then to the ampulla of vater, the area in the duodenum where the common bile duct drains into the small bowel. The second method is performed by an interventional radiologist and often happens only after adequate drainage has been demonstrated through a transcutaneous, transhepatic tube. The placement of biliary tubes and stents can be done as an outpatient procedure but may require overnight observation to ensure adequate drainage and sometimes requires antibiotics for temporary fevers and chills due to manipulation of the bile ducts and possible infection.

Biliary stents are either temporary, plastic ones, which have to be exchanged every 3 months, or permanent, metallic stents that are not meant to be exchanged. Metallic stents are often larger in diameter and keep the duct open longer, which means a lower rate of recurrent obstruction.[6] Metallic stents should be considered for patients with a life expectancy of at least 6 months. Their median patency rate—how long they remain open—is 8-10 months. The disadvantages of metallic stents are their cost and the difficulty in removing them once placed. There are ways to open these stents if they do become clogged, including placing a stent within the stent. I have found that if I have metallic stents placed in my patients, they have fewer readmissions to the hospital for biliary stent blockage than with plastic stents.

NUTRITION

One aspect of care that can be particularly frustrating for cancer patients and their caregivers is nutrition. Patients may not feel like eating or may feel full as soon as they start eating. Patients may lose weight despite a high caloric intake. I typically tell patients to eat whatever they like to eat. In Michael's case, it was Spaghettios. It makes very little sense to place any sort of restrictive diet on patients with pancreatic cancer, who are likely to lose weight if they reduce their caloric intake.

However, some consideration should be given to limiting excessive consumption of concentrated sugars, to avoid difficulties in blood sugar control, and of high-fat foods, to avoid poor absorption of nutrients in the gastrointestinal tract. Frequently I will have a patient who is losing weight because of carefully not eating anything with sugar, due to their diabetes, or who is afraid of "feeding the cancer," or who is on a BRAT diet (bananas, rice, applesauce, toast) because of diarrhea. Restrictive diets are sometimes necessary for symptom control, but it is far better to increase a patient's insulin dose or pancreatic enzyme dose than to limit food intake.

Patients will often ask about "starving the cancer" because they have read about studies on it, but I don't think this applies to patients with advanced cancer, who are often already not eating enough food.

Some patients may be limiting their food intake because of physical problems such a gastric outlet obstruction, in which the cancer is obstructing the normal flow of food from the stomach into the intestines, or due to ascites, which is fluid in the abdomen pushing on intestines. Some patients suffer from an anorexia-cachexia syndrome, in which patients have decreased appetite and have fat and muscle wasting despite caloric intake. This has something to do with cytokine production and alterations in metabolism, and it is complicated by depression, pain, malabsorption, and nausea.

Small doses of steroids or progestational drugs are sometimes used to stimulate appetite. There is an increased concern for blood clots with the use of megestrol (Megace). Dronabinol (Marinol), a synthetic version of delta-9-tetrahydrocannabinol, which is an active agent in marijuana, is sometimes used to treat nausea and stimulate appetite.[7] I have used these agents with variable success.

Another nutritional challenge for people with pancreatic cancer is pancreatic insufficiency. Pancreatic cancer affects the production of pancreatic enzymes, such as amylase, lipase, trypsin, and chymotrypsin, which help in the digestion and absorption of food. Malabsorption of nutrients can lead to weight loss, steatorrhea (greasy, floating stools), diarrhea, abdominal bloating, gas, and pain. Pills containing replacement pancreatic enzymes are available. They are dosed by their lipase content. Enzymes can be dosed by fat content of food or by weight, but I find it simplest to start with 2-3 tablets with meals and 1-2 tablets with snacks and then increase the dose by using symptoms as a guide. Up to 6 capsules at a time may be needed. Enzymes should be taken with all meals and snacks and should be taken whole. Taking the enzymes spaced out throughout the meal instead of all at the beginning of the meal can also be helpful. Acid suppression medication such as H2 (histamine) blockers

(Zantac, Pepcid) or proton pump inhibitors (Prilosec, Nexium, Protonix) can make the enzymes more effective by decreasing their breakdown by stomach acid.[8] Sometimes a change in formulation or brand can also improve symptoms. Enteric-coated formulations are typically recommended to protect the enzymes from breakdown by stomach acid. However, some patients have better symptom control with a preparation that does not have an enteric coating and should be prescribed with acid suppression to avoid degradation. Many pancreatic enzymes have been taken off of the market because the FDA has mandated that all pancreatic enzyme products obtain FDA approval to ensure effectiveness, safety, and manufacturing consistency. I have seen patients mistakenly take their enzymes at bedtime or several hours after a meal, which really defeats the purpose of providing pancreatic enzymes to help digest food. The quantity of these pills can be cumbersome for patients, but if taken correctly can help with symptom control, nutrition, and weight maintenance.

MALIGNANT ASCITES

Ascites is an abnormal accumulation of fluid inside the abdominal cavity. Malignant ascites is the accumulation of fluid inside the abdominal cavity due to cancer. The peritoneum is the membrane that lines the abdominal and pelvic cavity and surrounds the abdominal organs. The ascitic fluid fills in around the bowel and abdominal organs within the peritoneum. The fluid is usually free-flowing, but over time it can become loculated, or settled into pockets. Plasma, a component of blood, flows into the abdominal spaces as it leaves blood vessels and the lymphatic system, but in ascites it does not properly return to the blood vessels, resulting in increasing abdominal fluid and distension, or stretching.

Most often, ascites is a result of cancer cells in the abdominal cavity upsetting the normal balance. Although this cannot always be proven with pathology tests, it is often presumed. Cancer cells also may release inflammatory factors or block lymphatic drainage. Other times, ascites is not caused by cancer cells in the cavity or the linings in the cavity but because of reverse pressure in the vascular system. This might occur when the portal vein near the liver is narrowed due to cancer or a blood clot. The portal vein drains blood from the bowels into the liver (see Figure 8.1). Vascular pressure imbalance can also occur when there is enough cancer in the liver to cause back pressure into the same drainage system. Another explanation is that the albumin, or protein, levels in the blood may be low due to decreased function of the liver or due to poor nutrition. The low level of protein in the vessels makes it difficult for the fluid to stay in or return to the vessels.

The increasing distension in the abdomen caused by ascites can in turn cause pressure on the diaphragm, resulting in shortness of breath. It can also put pressure on the stomach or intestines, leading the patient to eat less or causing nausea, vomiting, or heartburn. Symptoms may also include swelling in the legs or feet, resulting in decreased mobility.

Unfortunately, ascites carries a poor prognosis, and survival is often measured in weeks after its occurrence. However, this is not always the case, especially if the patient has not received prior treatment and shows a response to therapy. I have had patients with pancreatic cancer and colon cancer for whom chemotherapy decreased the size of their tumors and reduced their ascites. When this occurs, it is usually early in the course of the cancer. I also had a patient with pancreatic cancer whose extensive liver tumors responded to therapy but whose ascites did not respond. Generally, ascites occurs at later stages and does not respond to chemotherapy.

The goal of any therapy or procedure to reduce ascites is to improve comfort. The mainstays of therapy for ascites are diuretics, or "fluid pills," and therapeutic paracentesis, which is a procedure that involves introducing a needle into the fluid space and draining some of the fluid (see Figure 8.1).[9] Diuretics are more likely to work if the ascites fluid is free-flowing and the result of pressure on the drainage into the liver, such as with extensive liver metastases. Diuretics are less likely to work if the ascites is due to cancer cells within the

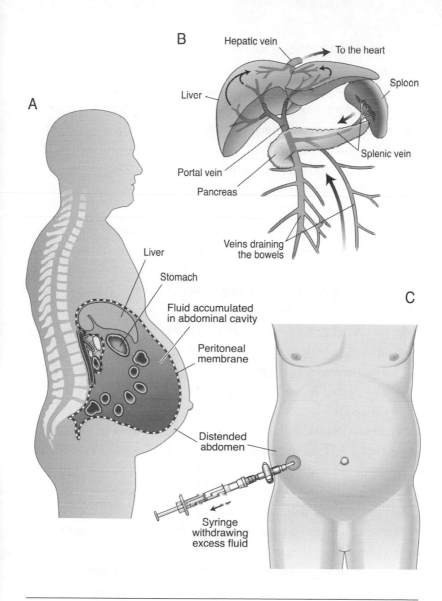

Figure 8.1 (*A*) Malignant ascites, an abnormal accumulation of fluid around the organs in the abdominal cavity that results from cancer cells in the abdomen. (*B*) Ascites can also result from tumors in the liver or clots in the main vein to the liver (portal vein) which increase resistance to the flow of blood and fluid draining from the bowels. The increased back pressure makes it difficult for the fluid to drain back through the venous system to the portal vein and into the main vein to the heart. (*C*) Paracentesis, the introduction of a needle into the fluid-filled space to withdraw the fluid.

abdominal cavity. Dietary salt restriction is helpful when diuretics are used.

Repeated palliative paracentesis (draining the fluid with a needle) is often required. The fluid usually reaccumulates, requiring the procedure to be repeated every ten days or so. The disadvantages of paracentesis include repeated visits to the treatment center, loss of protein over time, decrease in blood pressure, dehydration, risk for peritonitis (inflammation or infection of the peritoneum) or injury to the intestines.

Peritoneo-venous shunting, a procedure to shunt the fluid from the abdomen to the vessels is not typically a viable option for patients with gastrointestinal cancers, because given their poor prognosis, the benefits do not outweigh the risks. If portal vein narrowing is the cause of ascites, a portal vein stent can be attempted, but the data on this procedure are limited to case reports and case series with small numbers, so we do not know how useful it may be.

Physicians are increasingly turning to peritoneal catheters, tubes that are inserted in the patient's abdominal cavity and left in place to drain externally to a pouch or bottle, allowing the patient or a caregiver to drain the fluid periodically. Advantages to an indwelling catheter include decreased introduction of needles into the abdominal cavity and decreased frequency of visits to the treatment center. Also, smaller amounts of fluid can be withdrawn more frequently. This may help mitigate the dehydration that occurs from repeated draining of a large volume of fluid, which can lead to low blood pressure and poor blood flow to the kidneys. It is not known whether inserting a catheter from the onset of ascites improves overall quality of life measures for patients. Some of my colleagues are currently opening a study that asks this question. Potential downsides of indwelling catheters can be pain, bleeding, bowel perforation (a hole in the intestines), infection, leakage, blockage, and dislodgement. A recent review reported a low infection rate of 5.9 percent but a blockage rate of 37 percent among a variety of catheter types.[10]

GASTRIC OUTLET OBSTRUCTION AND SMALL BOWEL OBSTRUCTION

Cancer near the bowels can also result in bowel obstruction by a tumor, making it impossible for the person to eat or drink. Symptoms of obstruction in the gastrointestinal (GI) tract include persistent nausea, vomiting, bloating, abdominal pain, and constipation. Sometimes these obstructions are partial and can be reversed with conservative measures such as bowel rest and placement of a nasogastric tube. "Bowel rest" is achieved by not feeding the patient anything by mouth. A nasogastric tube goes in the nose and down into the stomach in an attempt to empty the upper GI tract and relieve pressure while the obstruction improves. Octreotide treatment may be useful.[11] Octreotide is an agent that can reduce secretion of fluids by the intestine and pancreas and can inhibit the action of certain hormones.

On occasion, surgical management is done to bypass a bowel obstruction. Unfortunately, in most cases, especially further along in the course of a patient's cancer, surgery is not an option. The disease is often too extensive. Bypassing one area does not solve the issue, because usually multiple areas of bowel are involved and therefore a single bypass procedure is often futile and the risks of complications from surgery far outweigh any potential benefit.

While surgical bypass is appropriate for a small number of patients, physicians are increasingly using enteral stents, which are usually placed by endoscopy directly into the GI tract. An enteral stent is a stent placed in the gastrointestinal tract to open up blockages to allow for the passage of food contents.

Gastric outlet obstruction occurs when the tumor blockage is at the level where the stomach drains into the duodenum (the first part of the small intestine). This is particularly common in pancreatic cancer because of the location of the pancreatic head, which sits right behind the stomach. Between 10 and 25 percent of patients with pancreatic cancer will develop a duodenal obstruction during the course of their disease. A stent can be placed across this obstruction to allow for the passage of food into the small bowel (see Figure 8.2). This will only be successful if there is not another blockage farther down in the intestines that will ultimately prevent forward flow of contents.

Success rates for correction of GI obstruction with a stent have been quoted to be in the 67–100 percent range.[12] However, the complication rate can be up to 30 percent, with a severe complication rate of 7 percent. Complications include bleeding and bowel perforation. Compared to treatment by surgery, however, patients treated with stents have fewer serious complications, less intensive care unit time, and shorter hospitalizations. Some later complications, such as stent dislodgement or clogging of the stent, can certainly impair a patient's quality of life. Because of these complications, patients with enteral stents often require dietary modification. In general, enteral stents are most useful for patients with limited survival prognosis.

Even temporary loss of normal bowel function often creates a very difficult time for patients, their families, and their physicians. There is a place for parenteral nutrition, intravenous nutrition, when the circumstances may be temporary or the bowels cannot be used for some reason other than continued progression of cancer. The American College of Physicians published a consensus statement that advised against the routine use of parenteral nutrition in advanced cancer patients undergoing chemotherapy. When used in cancer patients with malnutrition, the increased risks should be considered.[13] Guidelines put out by the American Society of Parenteral and Enteral Nutrition (A.S.P.E.N.) also support the view that parenteral nutrition is rarely appropriate for terminally ill cancer patients.[14]

It is extremely difficult to face the reality that when a patient begins intravenous nutrition, it will have to be short-lived and has its own sets of risks and complications, including electrolyte disturbances, infection, catheter-related complications, liver dysfunction, and fluid retention. Family members often feel that if this form of nutrition is not used or must be discontinued they are "starving" their loved ones. I am the first to admit that I have signed many orders to

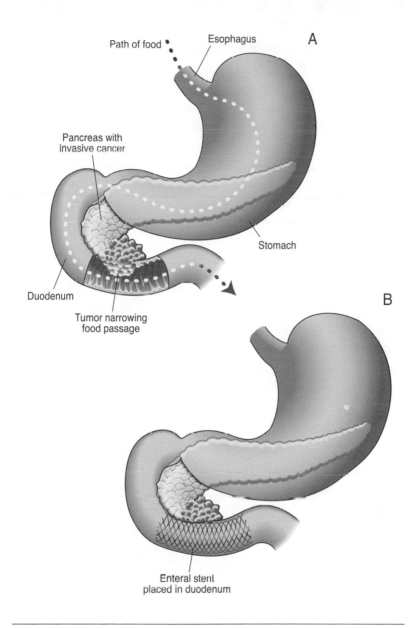

Figure 8.2 (*A*) Tumor pressing on the duodenum (the first portion of the small bowel). (*B*) An enteral stent in place holding open the duodenum to allow passage of food.

initiate intravenous nutrition, especially for patients who have re-mained active in their regular activities and have preserved a high performance status. Some studies suggest that patients with good performance status may benefit from parenteral nutrition.[15] The truth is that the use of parenteral nutrition in late-stage cancer pa-tients is controversial, and its use is unlikely, in the case of progres-sive pancreatic cancer, to improve outcomes significantly. Nonethe-less, many patients will receive this therapy because they and their families feel very strongly that they wish it. In my experience, the nutrition is typically administered for a few weeks to a couple of months near the end of life.

HOSPICE

This leads us to the topic of hospice. Hospice care is meant for the time when treatment for the cancer can no longer help. Hospice provides treatment to help relieve disease-related symptoms, not to cure or even slow the disease; its main purpose is to improve quality of life. The patient, family, and doctor decide together when hospice care should begin.

Hospice care can be provided in the home or in an inpatient hos-pice facility. An interdisciplinary team, including nurses, social work-ers, home health aides, physicians, and others focus on all forms of symptom management, emotional support, and spiritual support. Hospice will provide support for control of pain, nausea, bowel prob-lems, shortness of breath, nutritional issues, and many other medical problems.

One advantage of hospice care is that it is available twenty-four hours a day. Patients do not have to travel to see their physician. As the goals of care are focused on comfort, it helps avoid unwanted hospitalizations and treatments. It can mean a reduction in costs to patients and a comprehensive support system to address patients' and families' emotional and spiritual needs. The goal of hospice care is to help patients be comfortable while allowing them to stay in control and enjoy life and the people around them.

I have had very positive experiences with patients and their families who received hospice care. Often they felt that they were finally getting the comprehensive care they needed to cope during the final stage of the patient's life. I have also had patients who chose hospice over antitumor therapy from the beginning, at the time of their cancer diagnosis, and who lived well for many months. I have known families who started home hospice services but discontinued them, finding that the program didn't provide as much close daily care as they had expected.

Inpatient hospice facilities take full care of the patient around the clock, but family and friends are welcome at all times. An inpatient hospice may be appropriate when a patient's remaining time is expected to be short and symptoms are felt to be better addressed by an inpatient team of providers. Hospice does provide respite care—short-term full-time care to give the primary caregiver a rest. An inpatient hospice program can also provide short-term inpatient services to stabilize symptoms that have been difficult to manage in the patient's home. All hospice programs also provide bereavement care.

Depending on the individual's insurance, out-of-pocket costs for patients may be less while enrolled in hospice than in standard care under the guidance of the patient's oncologist. Once enrolled in a hospice program, the financial responsibilities of testing and therapies typically fall onto the hospice agency. Policies on certain aspects of care, such as artificial nutrition, blood transfusions, and paracenteses (extraction of unwanted fluid from the body), vary among hospice programs. Some patients feel that they would benefit from what a comprehensive hospice program has to offer but are concerned about limiting their access to such therapies, so these policies are something to think about when choosing a hospice program.

A number of hospices now offer "open access hospice," allowing more assertive types of treatment. This is more "liberal" than the traditional hospice philosophy. Certain therapies, such as blood transfusions and artificial nutrition, may be continued as long as they are palliative (improve symptoms). In some cases, this may include chemotherapy or radiation treatments. The benefit of open access hospice programs is that patients can get "aggressive" care along with comprehensive hospice care. However, such therapies are expensive for a hospice to support, so each case must be considered on an individual basis. While, as a community, oncologists feel that hospice services are underutilized and that patients nearing the end of life are probably overtreated, the individual patient's circumstances, goals, and fears have to be addressed in the overall decision about whether to use hospice, which program to choose, and which therapies to employ among those permitted in the program.

Unfortunately, in most cases, advanced cancers are incurable. When the diagnosis is received, one of the options open to the patient is hospice, begun immediately or begun after other types of care. Choosing hospice is not choosing death. Rather, it allows the patient control in how he or she will live the remaining time.

9

A New Approach to Living

THE MEDICAL SITUATION CHANGES . . .
AND CHANGES AGAIN

When my scan results showed some improvement in early 2008, I began to feel I might be able to hold on for a while. I do not remember being particularly hopeful. I think I said to myself, "This gives me a bit more time." In truth, I just accepted what was happening without thinking all that much. I did not want to get my hopes up.

By the middle of 2008, my condition was more stable and I was eager to do more. I planned a series of trips, thinking this might be the last time I would be able to visit some of these places. Ultimately, I found that I had bitten off more than I could chew. I wanted to go with Beth to Amsterdam and northern Italy, to Lake Como, in September, and I also planned a trip with my sister Laurie to Paris for her birthday in December. After doing much of the planning and even getting the air tickets, I finally decided that it would be too much to try. Beth did not want me to risk it, and I wasn't yet strong enough to do this on my own. Although I wanted to travel to Paris with my sister, where we had lived with our parents, Paris in December might have been brutal for me.

115

However, one trip that I did plan and that I insisted on taking was to New Zealand, to visit my youngest son, who had come to West Virginia with his family in April 2008. Beth was unhappy about my going but eventually agreed to come with me because she felt I would be safer if she were along. This was true. We took many precautions for the trip. We decided to travel business class with frequent flyer miles, so the trip would not be as exhausting. We stopped in Seoul, Korea, and Auckland, New Zealand, for two nights in hotels after the two long flight legs from Washington. We wore gauze masks inside the plane. I corresponded with two oncologists in New Zealand who specialized in pancreatic cancer, in case immediate care was necessary while we were there. We had had our flu shots, and it would be summer in New Zealand. Still, some might say this was risky, and, as it turned out, perhaps it was.

In February 2009, Beth and I made the long trip. My scans had been good for quite some time and my CA19-9 had been in the normal range for many months. At the time, I was considering stopping all chemotherapy, and, in fact, after the trip I had only one more session before taking a "chemo holiday" for a number of months.

I loved going to New Zealand, but I have to admit I was weak and still very dependent on Beth to care for me. It was not an easy trip. I was immune-compromised because of fourteen straight months of chemotherapy, so I was vulnerable to infection. During the visit, I did become ill. A local doctor had no answers as to what the cause of a rash on my hands, fever, and chills might be. Dr. Le had prescribed some antibiotics for me to take along, just in case, and she e-mailed Beth that I should take them. I felt better until they ran out, which was just about when we returned to the States. The fevers and teeth-rattling chills returned, along with a rash all over my front and back. This baffled everyone who looked at me.

We called our family doctor. He was not available immediately, and speed was vital, so I saw his colleague in the practice. We found it difficult to believe her diagnosis of Rocky Mountain spotted fever.

This is a tick-borne disease, but I did not remember ever being bitten. Nevertheless, a blood test proved her correct. It was great detective work. Where I contracted it remains a mystery. Luckily, excellent doctoring thwarted a potentially dangerous illness.

Another example of illness happened more recently. I felt a pain in my chest during one of our trips to Baltimore, so we stopped at an ER along the way. I was given prompt treatment and every possible test to rule out a heart attack or a pulmonary embolism. Fortunately, neither of these was the cause. After being examined by three doctors, I was admitted for observation. We thought this was ultra-cautious. The next day I was released and we continued on our way to Hopkins. Paula, my oncology nurse, on hearing of my chest pain, asked me whether I had been doing any unaccustomed exercises. I thought about that and the answer was yes, I had shoveled snow a couple of days before. Paula suggested a heat pad on my chest. The pain evaporated within a day. I recount this not to fault the doctors—they did the right things—but to point up the need to look at what is going on with your health from every angle.

The lesson from both of these examples is to stay on top of and investigate what is happening in your body, lest a small problem become more serious or even life threatening. It is also a good idea to be very cautious in placing yourself unnecessarily in potentially risky situations.

After our return from New Zealand, the scans in March and May of 2009 continued to show that the cancer was stable. The radiologist, world renowned, could not tell whether he was seeing very small tumors or simply scar tissue. There had been no change for eight or nine months, counting back from May 2009.

Dr. Le proposed a chemo break. Beth and I accepted readily. We were both happy. I had been on chemotherapy for more than a year, since December 2007. My bone marrow was depleted by the treatment, but the chemo had done its job. There was nothing more to knock down.

At the same time, Beth and I were realistic. We understood that this chemo holiday might be brief. Stage IV pancreatic cancer is not thought to be cured by chemotherapy and almost invariably returns.

I had a relaxing summer. We continued to live in the little house we had moved to after diagnosis, Green Hill Cottage. The end of summer is a magical time in West Virginia. I would sit in my favorite chair on the sun porch looking out at our neighbor Mr. Sowers's five horses grazing next to our fence. It was peaceful. I was pensive and content.

I had been off chemo for seven months, longer than anyone expected. My scans had showed essentially no changes for over a year, since mid-2008.

However, this changed in the fall of 2009. My CA19-9 level began to inch up and soon was above the normal range. Something was happening inside. A scan confirmed that there was again cancer activity in my liver.

AN EVOLVING APPRECIATION
OF END-OF-LIFE ISSUES

The prospect of beginning chemo for a second time focused my thoughts again. I wondered whether I had done everything I should have during the seven months off treatment. I think I had simply been hoping that the hiatus would go on forever. Dr. Le and I had started writing this book, but otherwise I had just enjoyed my time without chemo.

I thought of Patrick Swayze, the actor who had fought pancreatic cancer by continuing to do what he wanted, acting and living life on his own terms, as he defined them. I did not agree with his focus on working, since what he was doing seemed so strenuous. I did not think it was the best way to fight the illness, but I admired his determination to do what was meaningful for him.

We talked over with Dr. Le what was happening. I had made plans with my best friend, Peter Spalding, to take a cross-country road trip in September and was looking forward to this. Although I could have made this trip, I knew that it would not have been much fun with the prospect of beginning chemotherapy again hanging over me.

The day after seeing Dr. Le for the first time in six months, I decided to start chemo again.

I began thinking about things I had put aside. I would need to review my will. I would have to tell my kids that I was going back on treatment. We would make once again the trips to Baltimore. We would wait for the scan results to tell us what was happening. Most importantly, I would have to face up to the issues of death, which I had managed to put out of my mind, unrealistically, for most of those seven months.

I wanted to put what was happening into context. I wanted to explore how I should approach living if my second time on chemo proved successful, or dying if the opposite prevailed.

NEW APPROACHES TO LIVING

Sometimes I am impulsive, as most people are, but mostly I am methodical. I like to understand what is going on. So, I started by reading.

Just as I resumed chemotherapy, the *New York Times* published an article by Henry Grunebaum,[1] a psychiatrist and professor of clinical medicine at Harvard. Grunebaum recounted his experience working with a fellow therapist, a man who was dying. Dr. Grunebaum described an exchange between the two of them. He wanted to understand what his friend might be able to teach him about dying. There were two parts to the answer he received. First, his friend counseled him to keep a sense of humor, which helps one get through all the things that have to be faced. The second piece of advice was to do, or to continue doing, something that gives life meaning.

I knew exactly what his friend was talking about. You are feeling bad enough already when you are terminally ill. Maintaining a sense of humor is important. It gives those around you permission to smile.

I remember joking with my dentist about whether it was a good idea to do a certain (rather expensive) procedure, given that I might not be around to enjoy it. I also remember joking with my sons about some of the indignities of coping with cancer. I think this helped to put them more at ease in talking with me about what was going on.

The second point is elaborated by Dr. Grunebaum in his article. He describes how his dying colleague continued to help others. Not only were others helped but also, at the close of life, the therapist gained satisfaction in still being valued.

I had talked with several people who had survived cancer for some time, even stage IV cancer. Here is what one of them wrote, someone who had been facing death for years:

> I believe in living life to the fullest every day for the time I have left . . . I count my blessings and I look for a silver lining in the darkest clouds. I try not to sweat the small stuff and I try to let things go that I have no control over. I am very fortunate to have a great husband as well as a group of supportive friends. I try to keep things as normal as possible at home. There are times I do things that I don't feel like doing, but I think that even though I might not be up to par there will be times in the future that I will really need my caregiver. I push my husband to do things for himself such as golf games and golf trips. It is very important for me that he have a life. I try to stay positive and not go to the dark side. It takes so much energy to get out of that hole of depression. I do have "pity parties" but I try to keep them few and far between.[2]

There is a lot to reflect on in these few sentences. These include being positive, focusing on what is important, and being concerned for others. These give life added meaning. Dr Le and I are writing this book to help other patients, doctors, and health professionals. For my part, I am also trying to understand fully what I am going through.

In his article, Dr. Grunebaum points to another source, Irvin D. Yalom, a psychoanalyst, professor, and author, who was helpful to him. Yalom's story "Travels with Paula" in *Momma and the Meaning of Life*[3] presents an achingly honest look at the dying process.

Paula came into Dr. Yalom's life as a patient with stage IV cancer. She became his teacher during her journey. Together, they explored what it means to die.

Paula offered a positive, coherent approach to facing the fear of death. It began to move me from where I was—satisfied with a simple leaving, free of pain—which is certainly acceptable, and is what most people would wish for, to an appreciation that there could be a little more.

After my diagnosis, I needed reassurance that my death would not be painful. That allowed me to go forward. After I resumed chemotherapy, eighteen months after my diagnosis, and seven months after stopping chemo, the reality of my situation returned with full force. This time, however, I wanted to move beyond what I had felt earlier about dying.

Here is what I take from the story of Paula:

- Within the physical limitations that cancer imposes, there are still many things you can do.
- Death is an ending of the known. There may be little joy in it and much sadness at leaving life behind, but it is a part of life that everyone, every single person, goes through.
- We might want death to come at a different time, not when so much remains to be done, but we do not have that option. We do not have that choice. We have to find some meaning in its happening now.
- There may be a better place to go to, or not. We do not know.
- Thinking less of yourself and more of your loved ones can be a great solace. Preparing them for this next step is the best and final gift you can give them. This is difficult because it means facing up to one's deepest emotions of love for others and bringing them to understand that it is all right for them to let go of you.

A New Approach to Living 121

Remember the story of the lady who wrote the letter to her family and friends to tell them how much they had enriched her life. Remember as well how she told them it was all right to let her go without feeling too bad. Remember that she assured each of them she was happy they had been in her life. This is the right thing to do, and it is something others can emulate. This is a gift to those being left behind. It gives meaning at the end of life.

We also see this attitude in the woman who tried to live life to the fullest but also to prepare her husband for her eventual passing.

The late stages of a terminal illness can be a lonely and deeply depressing time, not only for the person who is ill, but also for a spouse or partner. It is a gift to them to ease their experience of this transition, to make things better for them. It is difficult, because doing so requires focusing on their needs.

It is also possible to make a difference in the lives of strangers even as yours is ending. One can, if strong enough, say no to many less important tasks and immerse oneself in things that really matter: a partner, friends, children, and even, for the very few fortunate enough to retain sufficient strength, meaningful work.

One of the first blogs I read when I was diagnosed was that of Randy Pausch.[4] He is a role model and hero in the pancreatic cancer community. A professor at Carnegie Mellon University, he had been diagnosed with pancreatic cancer, had had the Whipple operation, and learned later that it had been unsuccessful. He raised the public profile of pancreatic cancer through his appearances before legislative committees in Washington, D.C., and on the major television networks. He recounted his experience and inspired millions with his book *The Last Lecture,*[5] about achieving childhood dreams.

A source of inspiration for me is to read the stories of survival on the Pancreatic Cancer Action Network[6] and Pancreatica[7] Web sites. Few as they are, some survivors do find their way to greater service to others. For example, Jennifer Peelman, a two-year survivor, decided to return to her original life's dream of entering the medical profession. Chris Calpace, a six-year survivor, founded, with his wife,

Road 2 A Cure, an organization dedicated to educating the public about pancreatic cancer and the need to fund research to find a cure. Jeffrey Ross, another six-year survivor, has spent the last four years working the PanCAN phone assistance lines, helping others with all the problems associated with a diagnosis of pancreatic cancer.

Jennifer, Chris, and Jeffrey are not typical. The more common experience for those with pancreatic cancer is to live only a short time after diagnosis. I had already exceeded that average time, and as I contemplated being back on chemotherapy, I wondered what would happen. Although hopeful, because of my previous experience, I was realistic; this might be the beginning of the end. I went through a period of melancholy.

Just before I learned that I had to go back on chemotherapy, I talked with a friend in Shepherdstown whom I will call Barbara, whose experience with cancer is much more typical than mine. Barbara had had breast cancer, which she thought she had licked. Unfortunately, it returned with a vengeance.

Barbara had less than a year to live when we talked. She knew then that she would die soon. She was an inspiration to me and many others as she moved through the last stages of her life and passed away in July 2010.[8]

She told me that she had never paid much attention to having mammograms or to self-examinations. There was no history of cancer on either side of her family. Her grandmother had lived to be 113, her mother 94. But in her complacence she was quite wrong. Barbara managed to win the first round against this cancer, but eventually, when she was 65, it came back and it had metastasized to her bones.

When her cancer returned, Barbara was told there was little that could be done. She had been clear for almost three years, and this prognosis came as a shock. She was told more than she wanted to hear, at that first meeting, about how long she might expect to live. She had asked the doctor for her prognosis, but when the reply came in terms of a specific number of months, it overwhelmed her. When she had first been diagnosed, at 62, she had had surgery within a week and been pronounced well. She had not had time to really focus on death, she said.

Now, for the first time, she was confronting the reality of having stage IV cancer. Barbara feared the painful journey she was about to undertake. She didn't want to die, but she accepted that she was dying. She told me that she had had a good life, children and one grandchild, and many good friends who truly cared for her. She had lived in many different places before finally settling in Shepherds-town, and loved the town and asked for nothing more than to die there. During her last years, even into her last year, she worked in the town, befriending all whom she encountered. She was stoic about leaving us, and only asked that it be with a minimum of pain. She was able to have a radiation treatment when the pain became too much. Otherwise, she relied on pain medicine. She entered an outpatient hospice program, living at home when she was able and at the home of a close friend when she was not.

Barbara's final journey is an inspiration and evidence that it is possible to die a "good" death even when one has a relatively short period of time to prepare for it. Most people are sad, even devastated, to leave their lives behind. Sadness is inevitable, but it is possible to depart this life with a sense of having done positive things.

I did not know what awaited me this time round. I wanted to be as strong as Barbara.

CONVERSATIONS WITH BETH

The week following my return to chemotherapy, Beth and I had a long talk. We were in Baltimore for my second treatment and staying at the hotel. It was late, we were in bed, and it was raining outside. Fall had come suddenly and it was a cold rain. Our room in Baltimore overlooked both the inner and outer harbors. We could see the old Domino Sugar factory sign in red neon across the water. The reflections of the lights were in the water. Baltimore seemed somber that night.

We had never talked much about what I wanted to say that night. After my diagnosis, I had focused on my will and other documents. We had talked a little about where I might be buried, but only a little. That decision is, of course, just as important as those recorded in the advance directive and other legal documents. Still, it is difficult to talk about, and we had left much unsaid.

That evening, I thought it might be time to talk more about this with Beth. We talked for a long time about the funeral. By the end of the evening, I believed we understood each other's wishes better. No decisions were taken, but we had laid the basis for the next talk.

Discussing what will happen after death is important, but not paramount, depending on the family's situation. Some people will be perfectly content to leave the decisions to their family. Others prefer to immerse themselves in the details. I found I was most concerned about clarifying what would happen before my death, not after.

Although I am squeamish even thinking about this, I have decided that a rapid autopsy should be performed and that my organs should be given to Johns Hopkins for research. This can be a contribution to medical science.

At the end of our talk, I felt we had accomplished the last thing that had to be done. I slept better that night.

Later that week, I began to think about something else that had been on my mind. What would happen to Beth after I was gone? I had thought about this off and on for some time. Beth is far more independent than I have ever been and I think she will be all right. I feel sad about leaving her after so few years together. I wonder, will she stay in West Virginia, return to Maryland, where she lived most of her adult life, or go back to North Carolina, where there is family? I do not know, even now. But, I wanted her to know that whatever she decides is okay with me.

However, we did not have that conversation until more time had passed.

Our life together has had its ups and downs. Often, I have been able to do the things I wanted, while Beth has not. I tried to think of things I could do to make her life easier and better, even at this late date. I needed to make more time for us and spend less time on things that did not matter.

10

Next Steps

The long duration of Michael's chemotherapy break was a pleasant surprise. This takes us back to the goals of care for pancreatic cancer, which are primarily the best quality of life for the longest possible time. I think the chemotherapy break was important for Michael, to get the chance to live without the constraints of being a patient. We knew when we paused the therapy that there was some risk that the tumors might be resistant to treatment with the same regimen in the future, but we took the risk. Certainly, in other cancers, such as colon cancer, patients can be re-treated with the same regimen if the reason for stopping it was not progression of disease or growth of tumors while on therapy. We did not pretend that the cancer would not grow back. Again, chemotherapy is not curative in pancreatic cancer, but it certainly can provide benefit to patients.

Fortunately, for the time being, Michael appears to be responding to the reintroduction of GTX. I think the sense of urgency to finish this book which we both felt was enhanced by the reality that his chemotherapy holiday was over. We anticipate that the GTX will run its course—that at some point it will stop working. I have recently had to discuss other options with one of my other pancreatic cancer patients due to progression of the disease while he was on GTX.

CHEMOTHERAPY RESISTANCE

Chemotherapy resistance means that cancer cells are no longer responding to the administered chemotherapeutic agents. Some patients have cancers that are resistant to chemotherapy from the beginning. Various mechanisms come into play that promote this resistance. While scans may not show remaining cancer cells, they exist. We know this because of the natural history of metastatic pancreatic cancer. While tumors may stabilize or shrink, they will eventually grow. Remaining cells have mechanisms for inactivating drugs (drug metabolism). In addition, when they develop the multidrug resistance phenotype (MDR), cancer cells can pump the drugs out of themselves (drug transport). They can also stop taking in the drugs. They counteract the damage to their genetic material caused by chemotherapy through repair mechanisms, or by other strategies, and rescue themselves from cell death (genetic regulation and repair). Drug resistance is one reason why response rates to second-line chemotherapy regimens (a chemotherapy regimen used after the failure of the first) are lower than those to first-line regimens. At every step in the treatment decision process, the question must be asked, Is the potential for risks likely to outweigh the potential for benefits? This is especially true if the patient did not respond to first-line therapy. Of course, the patient's performance status must also be taken into consideration.

SECOND-LINE
CHEMOTHERAPEUTIC OPTIONS

As I think about next steps for patients, I often take the same approach as with the initial treatment decisions. As we consider second-line therapies, the patient's clinical status is likely to be more tenuous than at the onset of treatment, given symptoms of disease progression and postchemotherapy effects. Because of continued effects on bone marrow, second-line treatment may be more difficult to tolerate, due to drops in white blood cell and platelet counts.

When the time comes, Michael and I will discuss, as we did previously: standard treatment options, available clinical trials, known but not rigorously proven therapies, and symptom management without anticancer therapy. The decision not to pursue therapy may be less difficult for patients and their families at this juncture if patients have had a decline in their status or have not responded to their initial therapy.

According to the National Comprehensive Cancer Network of the Practice Guidelines in Oncology, second-line therapy may consist of gemcitabine for those patients not previously treated with the drug.[1] Other options include capecitabine (an oral form of 5-fluorouracil [5-FU]) or intravenous 5-FU or a combination of oxaliplatin with either capecitabine or 5-FU.

These recommendations are based on a series of smaller studies and one large study, CONKO 003, which demonstrated a significant improvement in overall survival with the addition of oxaliplatin to 5-FU, called the OFF regimen.[2] The median survival time among study participants was 26 weeks in the OFF group as compared to 13 weeks in those receiving 5-FU alone. No data on prior response to gemcitabine was given in the study reports.

Data from a phase 2 trial performed at MD Anderson Cancer Center suggests that XELOX (capecitabine with oxaliplatin) is more likely to be effective in patients with a good performance status and whose cancer responded to first-line therapy than in patients who did not respond to their first therapy.[3]

Most oncologists, because they are familiar with the regimens, which are also used to treat colon cancer, will use either XELOX or FOLFOX as a second-line therapy for pancreatic cancer. FOLFOX incorporates the same drugs as OFF, 5-FU plus oxaliplatin, but in a slightly different schedule.

Other options include the use of oxaliplatin in combination with fixed dose rate gemcitabine, which is gemcitabine given over a longer intravenous infusion than the usual 30 minutes. Small studies suggest that there is a subset of patients with gemcitabine-resistant cancer who will respond to this regimen, and I have seen this in some of my patients.[4] The GTX regimen described in Chapter 4 was reported to have a 25 percent response rate in metastatic sites in study participants who had progressed on previous chemotherapy.[5] In absolute numbers, this is only 3 of a total of 12 patients.

Other drug regimens that are used based on small studies or on anecdotal evidence include various single-agent or combination regimens of gemcitabine, cisplatin, oxaliplatin, docetaxel, irinotecan, paclitaxel, nab-paclitaxel, and mitomycin. In general, response rates in second-line therapies are low and the responses are of short duration. These studies also have a selection bias, in that patients had to be well enough to enroll in a clinical trial, which, in the case of second-line therapies, is probably a minority of patients and the strongest patients.

CLINICAL TRIALS

While I think it is necessary to take every individual's circumstances and wishes into consideration when making treatment choices, a clinical trial should be considered if one is available and the patient has a good enough performance status to participate. Some physicians argue that investigational therapies should be considered as early as possible in the course of a patient's disease, as this is the point in the disease that it is most likely to show a response to therapy.

Clinical studies will continue to be necessary if we are to progress in the treatment of pancreatic cancer, but I sense that it is getting more difficult to find patients who have not already been exposed to multiple therapies and are motivated to try new agents. And only 2 percent of individuals who have experienced disease progression during a first-line study treatment enter another clinical trial. Of course, many potential study participants may be medically unsuitable for a particular trial, and it may be that patients with a limited life expectancy choose not to spend their time involved in a research study. Clinical trials can be burdensome, requiring travel to participating institutions and additional time commitments. Advantages of participation include access to agents that may not otherwise be available for the treatment of pancreatic cancer, and the opportunity to contribute to the development of treatments for future patients. A patient on one of my immunotherapy trials asked to be enrolled in a rapid autopsy study being performed at Hopkins. She wanted to contribute in any way she could, even knowing she would not personally benefit from the study. Of course, this is a highly personal decision, and study participation is not appropriate for everyone.

I have referred to the "phases" of clinical trials. Simplified, the phases of clinical trials are as follows: Phase 1 trials are designed to look at safety, doses, and schedules of new agents or new combinations of agents. Phase 2 trials are designed to look at safety and at signals of efficacy in a homogenous patient population, and they typically restrict the tumor type, stage, and number of prior therapies of the participants. Phase 3 trials are much larger studies that compare a new therapy usually to the "standard" therapy. A government Web site that lists clinical research trials is at www.clinicaltrials .gov.

I have found that most phase 3 opportunities for people with metastatic pancreatic cancer are testing first-line treatments and typically compare gemcitabine to gemcitabine plus a new agent. There is currently an open first-line phase 3 trial of gemcitabine versus gemcitabine with Abraxane (nanoalbumin-bound paclitaxel). Some of the benefits of the nanoalbumin formulation of paclitaxel are that it does not require as large an amount of steroids, used for the prevention of side effects. In addition, it may facilitate delivery of the drug to the tumor. Interestingly, this trial was in phase 2 when Michael was initially diagnosed, but it would not have had an opening for several weeks and he wanted to start treatment right away.

When considering participation in a clinical trial, patients and their physicians should remember that the new drug combination may prove no more effective than those already in use. Such combinations as gemcitabine with bevacizumab (a blood vessel formation inhibitor), gemcitabine with oxaliplatin (another chemotherapy drug), and gemcitabine with cetuximab (epidermal growth factor receptor inhibitor) proved no better than gemcitabine alone in their respective phase 3 trials, despite having produced promising phase 2 data.

Also, when a clinical trial is designed that is going to randomly assign participants to either the control arm (usually gemcitabine alone) or the experimental arm of the study (gemcitabine plus the experimental agent[s]), the concept of "equipoise" or the "uncertainty principle" must be applied. This is an ethical principle that holds that there is true uncertainty about which of the treatments is more likely to benefit the patient. As demonstrated by a number of phase 3 trials of pancreatic cancer treatments, the group receiving the combination therapy did not necessarily fare better.

While phase 3 trials are less commonly performed in the second-line setting, the CONKO 003 study in Germany comparing OFF to 5-FU, was one such study.[6] For a patient who has received prior therapy, a more common scenario would be the availability of a phase 1 or 2 trial.

WHAT'S HAPPENING IN RESEARCH ON PANCREATIC CANCER

The wording of this section is more technical than the rest of this book, but if you have pancreatic cancer you may hear about these research topics. Always ask your physician if you do not understand something relevant to your diagnosis or treatment.

The *Journal of Clinical Oncology* published, in its November 2009 edition, a special report: "Consensus Report of National Cancer Institute Clinical Trials Planning Meeting on Pancreas Cancer Treatment."[7] Special emphasis was placed on studying the following topics: *K-ras* pathway, cancer stem cell (CSC) signaling, and the tumor microenvironment.

K-ras

The molecular pathways in pancreatic cancer are extremely complex, and knocking out a single target is unlikely to result in significant clinical benefit. However, a majority of pancreatic cancers have activating mutations in *K-ras*, and targeting this pathway as part of an approach to inhibiting multiple signaling pathways is thought to be an important strategy.

Cancer Stem Cells (CSCs)

Another popular area of research is in the field of cancer stem cells. As opposed to the more differentiated or matured cells that form the bulk of cancer tumors, CSCs are a small subset of cancer cells that are more resistant to therapy and account for both tumor initiation and tumor growth, or repopulation. They are capable of both self-renewal and the generation of offspring cells that are more differentiated, which means they have acquired some characteristics of cells that have attempted to mature into pancreatic ductal cells. This process has been described by a Hopkins hematologic malignancies oncologist, Dr. Rick Jones, as not just targeting the dandelion weed but targeting the roots that lie underneath the surface that will repopulate the lawn. The "hedgehog" molecular pathway provides signals in regulating stem cells and is involved in maintenance and regeneration of tissues and the development of tumors. This pathway is being targeted by researchers with agents that inhibit these pathways.

Tumor Microenvironment

The third research target area that was identified in the NCI report is the tumor microenvironment. The tumor microenvironment refers to the components of the tumor other than the actual cancer cells that contribute to the propagation of the cancer. These components include but are not limited to the other cell types, blood vessels, immune cells, and other regulatory molecules.

The report also made several suggestions in response to the multiple phase 3 studies that produced negative results. Treatments that have passed phase 2 trials need to have a high likelihood of success before entering phase 3 testing. The recommendations the panel made for future phase 3 trials include closer attention to patient selection, agents to be tested, statistical designs, correlative science, and transition from phase 2 to phase 3. In terms of patient selection, enriching the participant cohort for a trial based on a predictive marker may improve response rates. An example would be the selection of patients with a particular mutation in their cancer for testing a specific therapy. The report also supports establishing uniform eligibility criteria across trials. Patients with localized unresectable disease should be studied separately from those with metastatic disease, due to differences in prognosis. Agents should be tested in a multitargeted approach based on scientific rationale, and new therapies may be considered before gemcitabine when they are more likely to show activity, given gemcitabine's limited benefits. The report supports the use of survival as a primary end point and suggests implementing phase 3 testing only after a robust signal from pilot studies.

Hereditary Considerations

Not mentioned in the NCI report but, given Michael's ethnic heritage, an area of research that deserves mention is the role of heredity in pancreatic cancer. Michael does not have a strong family history of pancreatic, breast, or ovarian cancer. However, some patients with Ashkenazi Jewish heritage have a BRCA genetic mutation. Michael has tested negative for the most commonly detected mutations. There is increasing evidence that tumors that have a BRCA mutation may be more sensitive to certain chemotherapeutic agents because the mutation affects the cell's ability to undergo homologous recombination, a process that is used by some cells to repair themselves from damage caused by chemotherapy. Platinum agents, such as cisplatin, and an investigational class of agents known as PARP inhibitors may be more effective in BRCA positive tumors. PARP is an acronym for poly (ADP-ribose) polymerase. PARP proteins can repair DNA damage and prolong the life of a cancer cell. BRCA positive cancer cells treated with these agents are subsequently impaired in two methods of DNA repair. While the evidence is not strong, some physicians lean towards using a platinum agent in patients with a family history of cancer or in patients of Ashkenazi Jewish descent.

Immunotherapy

I would like to briefly mention immunotherapy, as my personal research interest is in the use of immunotherapy for patients with gastrointestinal malignancies. The goal of agents that target the immune system is to boost the immune system's fighting cells' ability to recognize the cancer cells as foreign invaders, in the hopes that the immune system will help identify and eradicate the tumor. There are many classes of immunotherapeutic agents currently being studied. There is a growing interest in a class of agents, referred to as immune checkpoint inhibitors, that actually block signals that tell immune cells (T cells) to turn themselves off. Blocking the signals would result in enhanced activation of T cells. There are agents in clinical studies now that target several of these signal pathways, including a cytotoxic T lymphocyte antigen-4 (CTLA-4) antibody and a programmed death-1 (PD-1) antibody. There is increasing evidence that these agents are somewhat effective against solid tumors. The extent of their activity and their true clinical benefit is yet to be determined, given the early stage of their clinical development, but I am optimistic.

"Cancer vaccines" are designed to boost cancer-specific immune cells. It is likely that if cancer vaccines do show a clinical effect, especially as a single agent, it will be in patients with the lowest disease burden, such as those who have had a surgical resection of their cancer. If cancer vaccines show any impact on metastatic disease, it will likely be only in combinatorial strategies. The future holds interesting trial designs that will combine vaccines with immune checkpoint inhibitors, chemotherapy, radiation, and other targeted agents in various disease indications and stages.

I CANNOT SAY FOR SURE what Michael's next step after returning to GTX therapy will be; we will have to make that decision together. I can say that we will explore the potential avenues in some detail before making a decision. As usual, his functional status at the time will be critical in the decision-making process, and we will choose an individualized path that will take Michael's current goals and wishes into consideration.

11

What We've Learned from Our Experience

This book is written from our points of view and with our specific experiences in mind, but confronting the many issues that cancer brings is a personal, individual journey. What helps one person may not work for another. Synthesizing what we have written into some small, practical steps may help others to apply what we have learned to their own situations. The lessons described below were written by Michael and are followed in some cases by comments from Dr. Le.

The suggestions and observations in the categories below are not listed in any particular order of timing or sequence.

GENERAL GUIDANCE

Know your family's history of illness. Being aware of risk factors for diseases that might be inherited is sensible. I was aware of my family's history, but I never connected the dots. Arming a doctor with this information will help in making a diagnosis. It can lead also to a good discussion with children of the reasons to avoid smoking and to favor healthy eating habits.

137

Monitor your health. There are often simple steps you can take that may be critical to catching cancer in its early, more treatable stages. For example, have pap smears, colonoscopies, and mammograms as recommended. If something is happening in your body for which there seems to be no explanation, pursue it.

Look for a primary care doctor who will take the time to explain what he or she is doing and why. Although it is tempting, do not decide on your own which specialists to see. Consult your primary care physician for guidance.

Do not ignore unexplained symptoms. This is more difficult with pancreatic cancer because there are often no symptoms until metastasis has taken place. Act rapidly when there is anything atypical happening in your body.

Losing weight is not always a good thing, even if you are on a weight loss diet. Losing weight too rapidly may signal a problem. Losing it when not on a diet is, of course, a sure sign of a problem.

DR. LE: I certainly agree with Michael that individuals should have a heightened awareness of their family history and of changes in their bodies and health. Without a doubt, smoking should be avoided. That being said, most cases of pancreatic cancer are "sporadic," meaning that they occur in patients without a family history of pancreatic cancer and who do not have any of the classic risk factors. In addition, for pancreatic cancer, we do not have a proven method for screening patients. A colonoscopy every five to ten years increases the detection of early colon cancers that can be cured by removal, but nothing similar exists for cancer of the pancreas. We don't even know that a CT scan or other imaging test, performed two or three years earlier would have picked up a localized cancer. While it seems intuitive that it would have, there are countless stories of patients who within a year of their diagnosis of pancreatic cancer had CT scans that were negative. I also agree that unexplained symptoms should be investigated but would emphasize that they be truly unexplained. The range of possible diagnoses for the symptoms that might indicate pancreatic cancer is wide and, therefore, I think the recommendation I agree with the most is to have an internist or generalist physician that you trust and who welcomes your questions.

ONCE A SERIOUS ILLNESS IS SUSPECTED

When cancer, or some other serious illness, is suspected, there are important, early decisions that need to be made, like where and by whom you wish to be treated. Seek out doctors and hospitals with a record of accomplishment in treating the suspected or diagnosed condition.

Time is of the essence. Do not delay. Procrastinating or avoiding possible bad news increases the chances of a less favorable outcome.

Prepare for the first meeting with the oncologist. Although this may be difficult, given the circumstances, research the suspected condition or have someone else help with this.

If possible, bring another person along during appointments with any doctor. It is never easy to remember what is said; the other person can take notes. Two heads are better than one when it comes to thinking of questions to ask.

DR. LE: I think that Michael's advice to come to a visit armed with information is good advice for some. For others, the barrage of new information can be a bit overwhelming. For those individuals, the first visit can serve more as an introduction to pancreatic cancer, and return visits may be the time to ask specific questions. There are many reputable Web sites that carry basic information about pancreatic cancer or clinical trials. They include: www.cancer.gov., www.cancer.net, www.nccn.org, www.pancan.org, www.lustgarten.org,

www.pancreatica.org, www.pathology.jhu.edu/pancreas, www.onco
link.com, www.mskcc.org, www.mdanderson.org, www.ucsfhealth
.org, and the Web sites of other major cancer centers.

WHERE TO BE TREATED

The more common the type of cancer you may have, the more
likely it is that diagnosis and treatment can be done near your
home. The converse is also true. Pancreatic cancer and other
less common cancers are better treated at places that see more of
these kinds of cancer, and those places are fewer. It *can* make a
difference.

That said, there are myriad factors that can influence the decision
about where to be treated. Being near to home, in a familiar
place, is always appreciated for various reasons. Cost is important. However, if possible, a decision based on health considerations is likely to lead to a better health outcome.

A research and teaching hospital is often the right choice for more
complex situations. Even so, whether or not to take part in a research study is a complicated decision. Understand the pros and
cons about this before making that decision.

Throughout diagnosis and treatment, have someone or more than
one person with whom you can talk over these and subsequent
decisions.

DR. LE: I would venture to guess that in a high percentage of cases
the second diagnostic opinions obtained at more sophisticated medical centers serve to reinforce the first opinion. So, for patients who
are unwell, the trip, expense, and delay in beginning therapy of traveling to get care are not necessarily appropriate. There are competent,
caring, and experienced oncologists in most regions of the United
States. They are knowledgeable in the standard treatment options

and can often offer clinical trials. They are also trained to identify patients who are not likely to benefit from chemotherapy. Don't get me wrong; I believe in second opinions, and a trip to a major center may allow patients to consider more options including clinical trial participation. It may give them access to a multidisciplinary team of surgeons, radiologists, radiation oncologists, gastroenterologists, pain specialists, and medical oncologists that may have alternative opinions regarding certain aspects of care. At Hopkins, we have taken patients to surgery whose cancers had previously been deemed unresectable, and we have advised against surgery when, to us, a complete resection of the tumor seemed unlikely. We have placed biliary stents and performed pain blocks for patients who could not have had these procedures done in their local hospitals. Michael is convinced that he is alive today because he came to Hopkins, but I remind him that there are other patients who started off with other regimens, including gemcitabine alone, who have also done well.

SOME NUTS AND BOLTS OF TREATMENT

Stick to your treatment schedule. Missing chemotherapy, although it is sometimes unavoidable, lessens the effectiveness of treatment.

Consult your doctor before engaging in activities that might endanger your health.

Do not ignore the possible benefits of alternative, unorthodox treatments, but be cautious about investing much energy and money in them. They are usually unproven and reports of their value anecdotal.

Follow the advice of your doctor regarding medicines and of your treatment center's nutritionist concerning food and nutritional supplements. Discuss with them any alternative medicines or supplements you are considering taking.

Maintaining weight is often crucial in withstanding the rigors of chemotherapy. Limit weight loss by eating foods that appeal to you. Choose maintaining weight over eating "healthy."

Physical and psychological comfort is important. Control depression and pain with the help of modern drugs.

Make chemotherapy or any other form of extended treatment as comfortable as possible. For Beth and me, this meant finding a welcoming place to stay when we went to Baltimore for my treatments.

Remember that your treatment is also hard on your partner or caregiver, for many reasons. Ask for and accept help from others that might ease that person's load.

DR. LE: The goal of chemotherapy in metastatic cancer is the best quality of life for the longest time possible. Sticking to the dosing and treatment schedule is actually not the norm. Patients are very individual in their reactions to chemotherapy, and oncologists are trained to react to this variability. Doses and frequency of treatments often must be changed. It is important that the patient and the oncologist communicate to meet common goals that emphasize quality of life.

AFTER DIAGNOSIS, PREPARE FOR THE FUTURE

It helped me to think of myself as a manager who needed to think through what to do next. Maintaining as much of a sense of control as possible is important.

Part of not feeling out of control is to reestablish some of the normal routines in the house and around the house, when you are physically able to do so.

Prioritize the things you need and wish to do and be realistic about what you can do physically.

Putting my affairs in order was the most important thing for me. Putting affairs in order usually means bringing your will up to date and having advance health care directives, a health proxy, and a power of attorney.

Think carefully about the care you will want in the event of unconsciousness and an inability to express your own wishes. What is finally decided, with the advice of someone you trust, should be embodied in your advance directives.

In addition to doing those tasks that you can control and do in the short term, think about some reasonable goals for the future.

YOUR FEELINGS IN THE FACE OF CANCER

The statistics for pancreatic cancer are grim, but the ones you will read are mostly averages and are usually a year or two out of date. Advances in controlling cancer are made almost every day. You may be one of the more fortunate persons. There *are* success stories.

This is a good time to rekindle and strengthen relationships with family and friends.

Think about your partner, who is probably also your principal caregiver. The diagnosis is also life changing for him or her. One of the greatest gifts you can give that person is to understand this. Hard though it may be, take the lead to prepare that person for the difficult days ahead and for your death.

You will have many feelings that should be recognized and addressed. One that I struggled with was a tendency to feel that illness should lead to entitlement. There may be a tendency to take the caregiver for granted. It may take time to recognize individual feelings and admit to having them. The sooner this can be done, the better for all concerned. One way to do this is to talk to professional social workers and others about what is happening. They can help you recognize what you are feeling. Discuss your feelings with your caregiver and your doctor as well.

Be aware that you may have considerable anger about your situation and that it may become misdirected against your caregiver or partner or other family members. It may be difficult to recognize anger. It may come out in unusual ways, so it is important, again, to talk with your caregiver and/or a professional about what is going on in your emotions.

Your caregiver is under considerable, sometimes unbearable, pressure. Be aware of this and try to find ways to reduce this pressure.

The love of family and friends is crucial to most people as they cope with the reality of having cancer, especially when it is first diagnosed. That said, family and friends should be made aware that receiving visitors demands time and energy, which, in both patient and caregiver, may be in short supply. Sometimes it is better for the ill person to be alone. Most friends and family will understand and accept this if it is explained.

Rules should be established and discussed with all visitors coming for a part of the day or for a more extended stay.

Problems that may have existed in the marriage or in the relationship may be exacerbated by a diagnosis of cancer. Be prepared for these problems to emerge or become stronger. Seek help quickly if you do not come to a satisfactory arrangement.

Second marriages, of which there are more and more, often come with stepchildren, adopted children, half-siblings, ex-wives and ex-husbands, and so on, and so forth. This fact complicates family situations and interactions and requires even more thought and conscious decisions on how to address these complications than simpler families demand. Be clear with everyone that the person with cancer is making the decisions about treatment and other important issues.

The Web site CaringBridge can be an invaluable tool for passing information to friends and family.

DEATH

Although death is never easy to discuss, it is helpful to talk about fears with your partner, caregiver, family, and medical team. Something unknown is often something feared. Death awaits each of us. Learning more about it will make it less unknown.

Most people fear the physical pain that sometimes accompanies death. Advances in drugs to manage pain and the increasing prevalence of hospice care today have made pain less of an issue at the end of life.

Having more knowledge and understanding of how the body shuts down and how people die helps some people cope with death. There are many sources of information about this.

Objectives such as the ones listed below may give added purpose to those living with cancer:

- Keep a small measure of humor about what is happening; it will help those around you.
- Continue to do the things that were meaningful to you before your diagnosis, within the limits of your physical

ability. Most people will not be able to continue working and will not have the strength to begin new endeavors. Often, the best thing to do will be to seek to improve family relationships.

- Show concern and care for your loved ones, who are also experiencing great sorrow and are anticipating loneliness.

When you think about your life and what kind of a person you are, and about your spouse or other family members and close friends, you may come to see, as I have in my own life, that you might have done some things differently, that you might have (this is my own personal list) been kinder, less argumentative, less self-centered, more loving, and more generous. If this is true for you, and if you have the time and opportunity, try to improve on what you realize was not as good as it might have been. This will mean much to you and to the people around you who are going through this process with you even if, like me, you fall short of your hopes.

AND WITH THIS, we come to the end of this book. It will not be the end of the doctor-patient dialogue we started under such trying circumstances three years ago. We both hope that our dialogue will help you, as it has helped us in many ways, to come to grips with the important issues that are encountered in dealing with cancer.

Postscript

I n 2010, Michael was able to go off chemotherapy a second time, for seven months. In November, however, he resumed treatment. As of the date of publication, he and Beth continue to live in Shepherdstown. Dung continues to conduct clinical research, teach, and practice medicine at Johns Hopkins.

APPENDIX:

SUPPLEMENTAL INFORMATION

Development of Pancreatic Cancer

Cancer cells develop from normal cells after a series of mutations in their deoxyribonucleic acid (DNA) or genetic makeup. As cells divide to replace ones that have died, their blueprint for the formation of daughter cells is encoded in the DNA in hereditary units called genes. The DNA is passed from cell to cell. Genes provide instructions for the production of proteins that are necessary for the normal activity of cells. Cell division, or mitosis, is happening all of the time in the human body. During this process, it is not uncommon for errors to occur during the duplication or reading of the blueprint, and this results in mutations in the genes. People inherit some of these mutations from their parents, while others may be caused by environmental factors, such as smoking. However, most of the mutations do not result in cancer cells.

Cancer cells arise when a cell acquires a series of mutations that gives it a survival advantage, in that it no longer has the capacity to heed the signals that tell normal cells to stop dividing. Also, these cells are often arrested in their development and cannot mature into adult form to carry out regular cell functions.

There are two categories of genes that are often mutated into cancerous cells. Proto-oncogenes, the first category, are genes that have a normal function in cell division. One of these genes is the *ras* gene. When proto-oncogenes are mutated or defective, they can cause continuous signals to divide. This would be analogous to a stuck accelerator in a car. The second category of genes includes the tumor suppressor genes. *P53* belongs to this category. As the name implies, a tumor suppressor gene has a role in the suppression of tumors, which are the result of excessive cell division. A mutation in this gene can result in its inability to provide a negative signal to cell division. This would be analogous to a defective brake on a car.

The evolution of normal cells to malignant cells progresses through a series of mutations, which often correlate with the transition from premalignant growths to frank cancer. Some mutations are thought to occur early in the progression, such as those in the *K-ras* oncogene. *K-ras* mutations are present in a majority of pancreatic cancers and are found in early PanINs, precancerous pancreatic lesions, identifiable under the microscope by pathologists. Precursor lesions have disordered growth but have not acquired the capacity to invade and ultimately metastasize. Alterations in other tumor-related genes, such as *P53*, *DPC4*, and *BRCA2*, occur later in the progression to higher-grade PanINs and to pancreatic cancer.[1]

Treatment Approaches: Resectable Disease

Physicians classify tumors according to practical categories: resectable (operable)/borderline resectable, locally advanced/unresectable, and metastatic (spread to other organs). Classification and staging (stages are described in Chapter 2) of cancers are accomplished with the help of sophisticated imaging technologies. Multidetector computed tomography (CT) with three-dimensional (3-D) reconstruction is the preferred method to diagnose and stage pancreatic cancer. Accurate staging is critical to identifying when surgical resection is appropriate. High-quality imaging and an expert radiologist and surgeon can help identify which patients should have surgery but also, importantly, who should not undergo unnecessary surgery. These scans can detect metastatic disease and major blood vessel involvement. Involvement of certain vessels, such as the superior mesenteric vein (SMV) and the portal vein, does not rule out surgery, and these cases should be reviewed by specialized pancreatic cancer surgeons. Tumors are considered localized and resectable if there are no distant metastases, no evidence of SMV and portal vein involvement, and there are easily visible planes, areas of tissue uninvolved by cancer, around the celiac axis, hepatic artery, and superior mesenteric artery (SMA). Borderline resectable cases may have some degree of involvement of these vessels but may still be considered to be resectable.

In 2009, approximately 5,000 patients in the United States underwent a curative-intent resection of pancreatic cancer. For patients with a lesion in the head of the pancreas, the surgery is called a pancreaticoduodenectomy, popularly known as a Whipple, after Dr. Allen Oldfather Whipple, who perfected the surgery. The Whipple involves the removal of the pancreatic head, the duodenum, and part of the bile duct, with a subsequent reconnection of the bile duct, stomach, and remaining part of the pancreas to the small bowel. Patients with more distal tumors (those farther from the head) will have a distal pancreatectomy and often a splenectomy. Because of the location of the tumors and the blood supply to the distal pancreas and the spleen, they are often removed together.

The experience of the surgeon is critical to the outcome of these procedures. The goal for surgical treatment of pancreatic cancer is to complete an R0 resection, which means that the cancer was removed with no cancer left behind. An R1 resection denotes a margin of tissue in which cancer can be detected but only at the microscopic level by a pathologist, and an R2 resection denotes that the surgeon left behind obvious cancer, which is known as gross residual disease. Cancer centers that do many of these surgeries have been shown to have a much lower complication and mortality (death) rate than low-volume centers.

Despite controversy over the most appropriate perioperative (before or after surgery) therapy to increase long-term survival, the 5-year survival rates for patients with resected pancreas cancer remain 15–20%. The underlying principle behind perioperative therapy is that the additional therapy will target microscopic disease left behind, which we know exists because of the high recurrence rates. Some institutions favor preoperative therapy (neoadjuvant). Others favor postoperative therapy (adjuvant therapy). Some institutions routinely incorporate radiation, and others do not. While trials of different treatment regimens have been performed, the best median overall survival time is still in the range of 17–20 months. Recurrence typically occurs within the first 12 months. Rates of local recurrence (at the site of the pancreatic bed or original tumor) remain in the 35–60% range, while rates of systemic recurrence (at sites distant from the pancreatic bed) remain in the 80–90% range. While there is plenty of room for improvement, the data do support the routine incorporation of some sort of perioperative therapy.

Using adjuvant, after-surgery, chemotherapy is the norm. The standard adjuvant therapies are: (1) gemcitabine, (2) 5-fluorouracil/leucovorin (5-FU/LV), and (3) gemcitabine plus 5-FU-based chemoradiation. Some of the studies supporting the use of each of these therapies are listed in Table A.1 and discussed below. The median survival times were similar in all the studies; they ranged from 20.5 months to 23.6 months. Several studies support the proposition that adjuvant chemotherapy improves outcomes for patients.

ESPAC-1, a European trial, showed a benefit of 5-FU/LV over observation (meaning, no chemotherapy) (median survival 21.6 months vs. 16.9 months).[2]

Table A.1 Sample of Adjuvant Trials for Resected Pancreatic Cancer

Trial	Treatments	Median Survival
ESPAC-1	5-fluorouracil (5-FU)/leucovorin (LV) vs. 5-FU with radiation followed by 5-FU/LV vs. observation vs. 5-FU with radiation	21.6 vs. 19.9 vs. 16.9 vs. 13.9 months
CONKO-001	Gemcitabine vs. observation	22.1 vs. 20.2 months
RTOG 9704	Gemcitabine + 5-FU with radiation vs. 5-FU/LV + 5-FU with radiation	20.5 vs. 16.9 months (in patients with head of the pancreas tumors)
ESPAC-3	Gemcitabine vs. 5-FU/LV	23.6 vs. 23.0 months

However, the most recent trend in the United States is to use gemcitabine as the base for adjuvant therapy. Since gemcitabine has proven beneficial for metastatic pancreatic cancer, it makes sense that there would also be benefit in the adjuvant setting.

CONKO 001, another European trial, compared gemcitabine to observation in resected pancreas cancer.[3] This trial showed a statistically significant disease-free survival benefit of 13.4 months with gemcitabine versus 6.9 months (P < 0.001) for observation. "Disease-free survival" is the length of time after treatment during which a patient survives with no sign of disease. Gemcitabine also resulted in a trend towards improvement in median survival (22.1 months vs. 20.2 months; P = 0.06), a trend meaning a result that is noticeable but not statistically significant.

An American study, RTOG 9704, also supported the use of gemcitabine in the adjuvant setting. Both study arms received 5-FU with radiation, but one group received gemcitabine in addition and the other 5-FU/LV in addition before and after radiation.[4] The gemcitabine resulted in a trend towards improved survival (20.5 months vs. 16.9 months; P = 0.09). It should be noted that this analysis was limited to patients with tumors in the pancreatic head.

Finally, the ESPAC-3 trial compared 5-FU/LV to gemcitabine and showed no survival difference (23.0 months vs. 23.6 months; P = 0.39).[5] However, there were fewer treatment-related hospitalizations in the gemcitabine group (3.5% vs. 10%). In general, while gemcitabine is not vastly superior to 5-FU/LV, most oncologists are still favoring gemcitabine.

The role of radiation remains controversial. Radiation therapy is the use of high-energy rays to target cancer cells. It is a localized therapy directed at the site of the tumor. It is often given with radiosensitizing doses of chemotherapy, in which case it is called chemoradiation. Radiosensitizing makes the tumor more sensitive to radiation. Early studies (GITSG, EORTC) suggested a role for chemoradiation in preventing recurrence of cancer after surgery. These studies did not compare chemoradiation to chemotherapy alone.

The results of the ESPAC-1 trial actually suggest a detrimental effect for chemoradiation, but this trial was not definitive, because of some flaws in the trial design and because the manner in which the chemotherapy and radiation were administered was considered not modern.[6]

The RTOG 9704 trial also did not answer the question of the role of radiation, because both arms of the study received radiation.[7] The rationale for continuing the use of radiotherapy is that local recurrence rates remain high. The 23% local recurrence rate in RTOG 9704 is the lowest rate reported by this group of studies. At a minimum, chemoradiation is usually incorporated into the treatment plan if patients have cancer at or near the surgical margin, the edge of the surgical area.

A consensus statement presented in 2009 in the *Annals of Surgical Oncology* regarding adjuvant therapy concluded that six months of adjuvant chemotherapy with 5-FU/LV or gemcitabine should be the standard.[8] However, six months of adjuvant therapy consisting of 5-FU-based chemoradiation preceded by and followed by chemotherapy is an acceptable alternative. Additional studies are planned and ongoing. ESPAC-4 is comparing gemcitabine versus gemcitabine and capecitabine (an oral form of 5-FU). The open RTOG study 0848 is testing whether or not the addition of erlotinib and/or chemoradiation to gemcitabine provides a survival benefit.

Regarding neoadjuvant therapy, preoperative therapy, at this time the National Comprehensive Cancer Network (NCCN) panel recommends that neoadjuvant therapy in cases of clearly operable disease should not be standard and is best administered in the context of a clinical trial.[9] However, in patients with borderline resectable disease, the majority of NCCN centers prefer an initial approach of neoadjuvant chemoradiation. Borderline resectable disease usually has partial involvement of blood vessels, and while the tumor is not definitely unresectable, it would be extremely difficult for a surgeon to remove without leaving cancer cells at the surgical margin. The neoadjuvant therapy can shrink the tumors as a whole or kill cancer cells at the edge of the tumor, making it easier for the surgeon to remove the entire tumor.

Neoadjuvant therapy has several advantages. It allows for early treatment of micrometastatic disease (microscopic cancer cells have already spread to other organs). Therapy can be better delivered to a primary tumor that has all of its blood flow intact and has not been disrupted by surgery. In addition, patients may be able to tolerate therapy better before than after a major operation. Presurgical therapy could potentially improve the likelihood of a margin-negative resection (no cancer cells left at the surgical margin) and decrease rates of tumor regrowth at the site of the pancreatic bed. Most important, it may keep patients with an aggressive cancer from enduring a major operation that would not benefit them anyway. Patients who develop metastatic disease during this time interval are the very same patients who would have been found to have "new" metastases on their first postoperative scan. These metastases probably were present as micrometastases prior to the operation.

Treatment Approaches: Locally Advanced Disease

Approximately 40% of pancreatic cancer patients are diagnosed with locally advanced disease at the time of diagnosis. In locally advanced disease, cancer has not yet spread beyond the pancreas and regional lymph nodes but it is considered to be too extensive within the local areas to be operable. Locally advanced disease can be treated with either chemotherapy alone or chemotherapy and chemoradiation. Difficulties in enrolling patients in chemoradiation studies have contributed to a lack of data about it. In addition, study results have been contradictory (see Table A.2 and discussion following). However, chemoradiation is a conventional option for locally advanced disease.

Several studies of chemoradiation reported results several decades ago. One study (GITSG) compared 60 Gy of radiation alone versus 5-FU with 40 Gy of radiation versus 5-FU with 60 Gy of radiation.[10] The median survivals were 5.3, 7.0, and 7.6 months, respectively. Patients who received chemoradiation survived longer compared to those who received radiation alone.

In the FFCD-SFRO study from France, gemcitabine alone was compared with 5-FU/cisplatin-based radiation followed by gemcitabine.[11] The study reported a shorter survival in the chemoradiation arm (8.6 months) than in the gemcitabine arm (13 months, P = 0.03). The toxicity of this

Table A.2 Sample of Trials for Locally Advanced Pancreatic Cancer

Trial	Treatments	Median Survival
GITSG	5-fluorouracil (5-FU) with 60 Gy of radiation vs. 5-FU with 40 Gy of radiation vs. 60 Gy of radiation	7.6 vs. 7 vs. 5.3 months
FFCD-SFRO	Gemcitabine vs. 5-FU/cisplatin with radiation followed by gemcitabine	13 vs. 8.6 months
E4201	Gemcitabine with radiation followed by gemcitabine vs. gemcitabine	11.0 vs. 9.2 months

particular chemotherapy and radiation combination may have accounted for this outcome.

However, in a third study, E4201, gemcitabine in combination with radiotherapy did better than gemcitabine alone (11 vs. 9.2 months median survival).[12] Higher toxicity (grade IV) was more common in the combination arm. This study was closed early due to poor enrollment.

There are reasons other than the improvement in survival to consider chemoradiation. Chemoradiation of previously nonresectable tumors can result in the "downstaging" of the tumors to the degree that they become operable. However, this occurs in only 5% of cases.

Much about chemoradiation has not yet been studied. No trials have specifically addressed whether or not chemoradiation reduces the risk of blockage of the bowel or the bile duct. Chemoradiation may help with pain control. A period of chemotherapy followed by chemoradiation may be preferred to chemoradiation at the onset of therapy. A retrospective analysis of outcomes from the French study group GERCOR indicates that giving chemotherapy and then reevaluating before giving chemoradiation may be a useful strategy for predicting which patients are more likely to benefit from chemoradiation.[13] If a patient's disease metastasizes in a short amount of time on chemotherapy alone, they would be unlikely to benefit from radiation that is directed only at the pancreas and the surrounding area.

NOTES

Chapter 2 • What Is Pancreatic Cancer and What Are Its Symptoms?

1. A. Jemal et al., "Cancer Statistics, 2010," *CA Cancer Journal for Clinicians,* 2010, 60(5):277–300.

Chapter 3 • The Fight Begins

1. J. Brody, *Jane Brody's Guide to the Great Beyond: A Practical Primer to Help You and Your Loved Ones Prepare Medically, Legally, and Emotionally for the End of Life* (New York: Random House, 2009), pp. xviii–xix.

2. S. B. Nuland, *How We Die, Reflections on Life's Final Chapter* (New York: Alfred A. Knopf, 1994), pp. 224–233.

3. R. L. Fine et al., "The Gemcitabine, Docetaxel, and Capecitabine (GTX) Regimen for Metastatic Pancreatic Cancer: A Retrospective Analysis," *Cancer Chemotherapy and Pharmacology,* 2008, 61(1):167–175.

4. The Web address for CancerCompass is www.cancercompass.com.

5. Personal interview, September 2009.

6. The Web address for the Pancreatic Cancer Action Network is www .pancan.org.

7. The program I participate in is the National Familial Pancreas Tumor Registry, http://pathology.jhu.edu/pancreas/PartNFPTR.php.

Chapter 4 • The Initial Treatment

1. H. A. Burris 3rd et al., "Improvements in Survival and Clinical Benefit with Gemcitabine as First-line Therapy for Patients with Advanced Pancreas Cancer: A Randomized Trial," *Journal of Clinical Oncology*, 1997, 15(6): 2403–2413.

2. M. J. Moore et al., "Erlotinib plus Gemcitabine Compared with Gemcitabine Alone in Patients with Advanced Pancreatic Cancer: A Phase III Trial of the National Cancer Institute of Canada Clinical Trials Group," *Journal of Clinical Oncology*, 2007, 25(15):1960–1966.

3. R. Herrmann et al., "Gemcitabine plus Capecitabine Compared with Gemcitabine Alone in Advanced Pancreatic Cancer: A Randomized, Multicenter, Phase III Trial of the Swiss Group for Clinical Cancer Research and the Central European Cooperative Oncology Group," *Journal of Clinical Oncology*, 2007, 25(16):2212–2217.

4. T. Conroy et al., "Randomized Phase III Trial comparing FOLFIRINOX (F:5FU/Leucovorin [LV], Irinotecan [I], and Oxaliplatin [O]) versus Gemcitabine (G) as First-line Treatment for Metastatic Pancreatic Adenocarcinoma (MPA): Preplanned Interim Analysis Results of PRODIGE 4/ACCORD 11 Trial," *Journal of Clinical Oncology*, 2010, 28(15 suppl.): Abstract 4010.

5. R. L. Fine et al., "The Gemcitabine, Docetaxel, and Capecitabine (GTX) Regimen for Metastatic Pancreatic Cancer: A Retrospective Analysis," *Cancer Chemotherapy and Pharmacology*, 2008, 61(1):167–175.

6. R. L. Fine et al., "Phase II Trial of GTX Chemotherapy in Metastatic Pancreatic Cancer," *Journal of Clinical Oncology*, 2008, 27(15 suppl.): Abstract 4623.

7. Guidelines for the treatment of adult cancer pain are available from the National Comprehensive Cancer Network at www.nccn.org.

Chapter 5 • The Prospect of Death

1. G. M. Condon, Esq., and J. L. Condon, Esq., *Beyond the Grave: The Right Way and the Wrong Way of Leaving Money to Your Children (and Others)* (HarperCollins Publishers, 2001, revised edition).

2. Personal interview, September 2009.

3. Personal interview, August 2009.

4. J. Brody, *Jane Brody's Guide to the Great Beyond: A Practical Primer to Help You and Your Loved Ones Prepare Medically, Legally, and Emotionally for the End of Life* (New York: Random House, 2009).

5. B. Veysman, "Full Code," *Health Affairs*, 2005, 24(5):1311–1316, http://content.healthaffairs.org/cgi/content/full/24/5/1311. An excerpt from this article describes what happens with many people when they go to the emergency room. The excerpt illustrates the issues faced in an ER and what

the medical profession feels obligated to do to save your life. It provides graphic evidence of the importance of thinking very seriously about having a living will and health proxy.

> Full code is permission for a doctor to insert a tube into failing lungs, shock a fibrillating heart, and unleash a plethora of punctures, dissections, and exsanguinations on the human body. These interventions save lives and restore functioning for a small number of people. For many others, they take their final hours of pain, suffering, and death and stretch them into weeks, even months of agony as organs fail one by one while the brain can still experience anger, depression, and pain. Yet to give the lucky few patients a chance to recover, all patients are granted full-code status until their wishes can be verified through documents or conversation. (1312)

6. Personal interview, September 2009.

7. Brody, pp. 23–45.

8. R. A. Moody, Jr., *Life after Life* (Atlanta: Mockingbird Books, 1975).

9. S. B. Nuland, *How We Die: Reflections on Life's Final Chapter* (New York: Alfred A. Knopf, 1994).

10. Nuland, pp. 208–209.

11. E. Kübler-Ross, *On Death and Dying* (New York: Collier Books, Macmillan Publishing, 1969).

Chapter 6 • Balancing Hope and Truth

1. Information about advance care directives is available at www.aging withdignity.org and www.caringinfo.org/stateaddownload.

2. S. E. Bedell et al., "Survival after Cardiopulmonary Resuscitation in the Hospital," *New England Journal of Medicine,* 1983, 309(10):569–576.

3. E. Kodish and S. Post, "Oncology and Hope," *Journal of Clinical Oncology,* 1995, 13(7):1817.

4. J. H. Von Roenn and C. F. von Gunten, "Setting Goals to Maintain Hope," *Journal of Clinical Oncology,* 2003, 21(3):570–574.

5. P. A. Francis, "Surprised by Hope," *Journal of Clinical Oncology,* 2008, 26(36):6001–6002.

6. The following Web sites offer information and support for caregivers: www.sharethecare.org, www.cfad.org, and www.pancan.org.

Chapter 7 • Family and Friends

1. Personal interview, August 2009.

2. CaringBridge, at www.caringbridge.org, facilitates sharing of information and support among patients and families facing significant health challenges.

3. Personal interview, October 2009.
4. Personal e-mail, June 2010.
5. Personal e-mail, June 2010.

Chapter 8 • Managing the Symptoms of Advanced Cancer

1. N. Makrilia et al., "Depression and Pancreatic Cancer: A Poorly Understood Link," *Journal of the Pancreas,* 2009, 10(1):69–76; and D. P. Kelsen et al., "Pain and Depression in Patients with Newly Diagnosed Pancreas Cancer," *Journal of Clinical Oncology,* 1995, 13(3):748–755.

2. J. L. Cullum et al., "Bupropion Sustained Release Treatment Reduces Fatigue in Cancer Patients," *Canadian Journal of Psychiatry,* 2004, 49(2):139–144; and E. L. Moss et al., "An Open-Label Study of the Effects of Bupropion SR on Fatigue, Depression and Quality of Life of Mixed-Site Cancer Patients and Their Partners," *Psychooncology,* 2006, 15(3):259–267.

3. J. L. Lillemoe et al., "Chemical Splanchnicectomy in Patients with Unresectable Pancreatic Cancer: A Prospective Randomized Trial," *Annals of Surgery,* 1993, 217(5):447–455.

4. M. Kaufman et al., "Efficacy of Endoscopic Ultrasound-Guided Celiac Plexus Block and Celiac Plexus Neurolysis for Managing Abdominal Pain Associated with Chronic Pancreatitis and Pancreatic Cancer," *Journal of Clinical Gastroenterology,* 2010, 44(2):127–134.

5. A. Y. Lee et al., "Randomized Comparison of Low-Molecular-Weight Heparin versus Oral Anticoagulant Therapy for the Prevention of Recurrent Venous Thromboembolism in Patients with Cancer (CLOT) Investigators," *New England Journal of Medicine,* 2003, 349(2):146–153.

6. A. C. Moss, E. Morris, and P. MacMathuna, "Palliative Biliary Stents for Obstructing Pancreatic Carcinoma," *Cochrane Database of Systematic Reviews,* Jan. 25, 2006 (1):CD004200.

7. N. Gullett et al., "Cancer-Induced Cachexia: A Guide for the Oncologist," *Journal of the Society for Integrative Oncology,* 2009, 7(4):155–169.

8. V. Damerla, V. Gotlieb, and M. W. Saif, "Pancreatic Enzyme Supplementation in Pancreatic Cancer," *Journal of Supportive Oncology,* 2008, 6(8): 393–396.

9. M. W. Saif, I. A. Siddiqui, and M. A. Sohail, "Management of Ascites due to Gastrointestinal Malignancy," *Annals of Saudi Medicine,* 2009, 29(5): 369–377.

10. N. D. Fleming et al., "Indwelling Catheters for the Management of Refractory Malignant Ascites: A Systematic Literature Overview and Retrospective Chart Review," *Journal of Pain Symptom Management,* 2009, 38(3): 341–349.

11. C. Ripamonti and S. Mercadante, "How to Use Octreotide for Malignant Bowel Obstruction," *Journal of Supportive Oncology,* 2004, 2(4):357–364.

12. L. Larssen, A. W. Medhus, and T. Hauge, "Treatment of Malignant Gastric Outlet Obstruction with Stents: An Evaluation of the Reported Variables for Clinical Outcome," *BMC Gastroenterology,* 2009, 9:45.

13. American College of Physicians, "Parenteral Nutrition in Patients Receiving Cancer Chemotherapy," *Annals of Internal Medicine,* 1989, 110(9): 734–736.

14. D. A. August and M. B. Huhmann, "A.S.P.E.N. Clinical Guidelines: Nutrition Support Therapy during Adult Anticancer Treatment and in Hematopoietic Cell Transplantation," *Journal of Parenteral and Enteral Nutrition,* 2009, 33(5):472–500.

15. I. Chermesh et al., "Home Parenteral Nutrition (HTPN) for Incurable Patients with Cancer with Gastrointestinal Obstruction: Do the Benefits Outweigh the Risks?" *Medical Oncology,* Online First, Jan. 27, 2010.

Chapter 9 • A New Approach to Living

1. H. Grunebaum, "A Final Round of Therapy, Fulfilling the Needs of 2," October 6, 2009, *New York Times,* health section, D5.

2. Personal e-mail, November 2009.

3. I. D. Yalom, *Momma and the Meaning of Life: Tales of Psychotherapy* (New York: Harper Perennial, 2000).

4. Randy Pausch's blog is at http://download.srv.cs.cmu.edu/~pausch/news/index.html. •

5. R. Pausch, *The Last Lecture* (New York: Hyperion Books, 2008).

6. www.pancan.org is the Web site of the Pancreatic Cancer Action Network.

7. www.pancreatica.org, as its subtitle says, is devoted to "Helping Patients and Physicians Create Optimal Treatment Strategies."

8. Personal interview, August 2009.

Chapter 10 • Next Steps

1. National Comprehensive Cancer Network, "Pancreatic Adenocarcinoma," *Clinical Practice Guidelines in Oncology,* 2009, 5(1).

2. U. Pelzer et al., eds., "A Randomized Trial in Patients with Gemcitabine Refractory Pancreatic Cancer: Final Results of the CONKO 003 Study," *Journal of Clinical Oncology,* 2008, 26(20 suppl.), Abstract 4508.

3. H. Q. Xiong et al., "Phase 2 Trial of Oxaliplatin Plus Capecitabine (XELOX) as Second-Line Therapy for Patients with Advanced Pancreatic Cancer," *Cancer,* 2008, 113(8):2046–2052.

4. A. Demols et al., "Gemcitabine and Oxaliplatin (GEMOX) in Gemcitabine Refractory Advanced Pancreatic Adenocarcinoma: A Phase II Study," *British Journal of Cancer,* 2006, 94(4):481—485.

5. R. L. Fine et al., "The Gemcitabine, Docetaxel, and Capecitabine (GTX) Regimen for Metastatic Pancreatic Cancer: A Retrospective Analysis," *Cancer Chemotherapy and Pharmacology,* 2008, 61(1):167—175.

6. Pelzer, Abstract 4508.

7. P. A. Philip et al., "Consensus Report of National Cancer Institute Clinical Trials Planning Meeting on Pancreas Cancer Treatment," *Journal of Clinical Oncology,* 2009, 27(33):5660—5669.

Appendix • Supplemental Information

1. R. H. Hruban et al., "Progression Model for Pancreatic Cancer," *Clinical Cancer Research,* 6(8):2969—2972.

2. J. P. Neoptolemos et al., "A Randomized Trial of Chemoradiotherapy and Chemotherapy after Resection of Pancreatic Cancer," *New England Journal of Medicine,* 2004, 350:1200—1210.

3. H. Oettle et al., "Adjuvant Chemotherapy with Gemcitabine vs Observation in Patients Undergoing Curative-Intent Resection of Pancreatic Cancer: A Randomized Controlled Trial," *Journal of the American Medical Association,* 2007, 297(3):267—277.

4. W. F. Regine et al., "Fluorouracil vs. Gemcitabine Chemotherapy before and after Fluorouracil-Based Chemoradiation following Resection of Pancreatic Adenocarcinoma: A Randomized Controlled Trial," *Journal of the American Medical Association,* 2008, 299(9):1019—1026.

5. J. Neoptolemos et al., "A Multicenter, International, Open-Label, Randomized, Controlled Phase III Trial of Adjuvant 5-fluorouracil/folinic Acid (5-FU/FA) Versus Gemcitabine (GEM) in Patients with Resected Pancreatic Ductal Adenocarcinoma," *Journal of Clinical Oncology,* 2009, 27(18 suppl.), Abstract LBA4505.

6. J. Neoptolemos et al., European Study Group for Pancreatic Cancer, 2004, "A Randomized Trial of Chemoradiotherapy and Chemotherapy after Resection of Pancreatic Cancer," *New England Journal of Medicine,* 2004, 350(12):1200—1210.

7. Regine et al.

8. J. N. Vauthey and E. Dixon. "AHPBA/SSO/SSAT Consensus Conference on Resectable and Borderline Resectable Pancreatic Cancer: Rationale and Overview of the Conference," *Annals of Surgical Oncology,* 2009, 16(7): 1725—1726.

9. National Comprehensive Cancer Network, "Pancreatic Adenocarcinoma," *Clinical Practice Guidelines in Oncology,* 2009, 5(1).

10. Gastrointestinal Study Group, "A Multi-institutional Comparative Trial of Radiation Therapy Alone and in Combination with 5-Fluorouracil for Locally Unresectable Pancreatic Carcinoma," *Annals of Surgery*, 1979, 189(2): 205–208.

11. B. Chauffert et al., "Phase III Trial Comparing Intensive Induction Chemoradiotherapy (60 Gy, infusional 5-FU and intermittent cisplatin) followed by Maintenance Gemcitabine with Gemcitabine Alone for Locally Advanced Unresectable Pancreatic Cancer (Definitive Results of the 2000–01 FFCD/SFRO Study)," *Annals of Oncology*, 2008, 19:1592–1599.

12. P. J. Loehrer et al., eds., "A Randomized Phase III Study of Gemcitabine in Combination with Radiation Therapy versus Gemcitabine Alone in Patients with Localized, Unresectable Pancreatic Cancer: E4201," *Journal of Clinical Oncology*, 2008, 26(15 suppl.), Abstract 4506.

13. F. Huguet et al., "Impact of Chemoradiotherapy after Disease Control with Chemotherapy in Locally Advanced Pancreatic Adenocarcinoma in GERCOR Phase II and III Studies," *Journal of Clinical Oncology*, 2007, 25(3): 326–331.

INDEX

The letters *t* and *f* following a page number refer to a table or figure.

BRAT (bananas, rice, applesauce, toast) diet, 103
BRCA genes, 13, 37, 134—135, 150
Brody, Jane, 23, 52, 55, 57; *Guide to the Great Beyond*, 23, 55
bupropion, 80, 98

CA19-9 blood test, as marker for pancreatic cancer, 7, 13, 79
cancer: breaking the news, 16—17, 84—86; described, 60—61, 149—150; impact on marriages, 82, 144—145; need for second opinion, 21, 140; resistance to chemotherapy, 128; stages of, 11; vaccines for, 135—136; where to be treated, 3, 140—141
CancerCompass, 31
cancer stem cell (CSC), 132—133
capecitabine (Xeloda), 43, 129, 153
cardiac arrest, 67—68
cardiopulmonary resuscitation (CPR), 67
caregivers: need for support of, 73—74, 90, 142, 143, 144; and respite care, 113; responsibilities of, 5, 78, 82, 108. *See also* Beth
CaringBridge Web site, 77, 145
CBC (complete blood count), 48
celiac axis, 11, 150
cetuximab (epidermal growth factor receptor inhibitor), 132
Charbel, Saint, 59
chemoradiation, 151—155
chemotherapy: goals of, 19; options for treatment with, 39—49; resistance to, 128; as second-line treatments, 128—129
cholangitis, 102
cisplatin, 43, 130, 134, 154
Cleveland Clinic, 26

clinical research trials: in academic institutions, 45; necessity of, 130; new directions in, 132—134; phases of, 131, 134; prospective and retrospective, 46; uncertainty principle, 132
common bile duct, 12, 14f, 102
complete blood count (CBC), 48
CONKO 001 study, 152
CONKO 003 study, 129, 132
Consensus Report of National Cancer Institute Clinical Trials, 132
Coumadin (warfarin), 101
CPR (cardiopulmonary resuscitation), 67
CSC (cancer stem cell), 132—133
CT (computed tomography) scans: for diagnosis of pulmonary emboli, 100; Michael's, 13, 16f, 95; use of, in staging decisions, 150
cytotoxic T lymphocyte antigen-4 (CTLA-4) antibody, 135

death: and afterlife, 59; counseling about, 61—62; legal documents regarding, 54—57; patients' fears about, 61, 72—73
deep vein thrombosis (DVT), 100
depression and anxiety, 96—98
diabetes, 12, 16, 96, 103
diuretics, 106, 108
DNA (deoxyribonucleic acid), 18, 135, 149
DNR (do-not-resuscitate) order, 67
docetaxel, 130
Doppler ultrasound instrument, 100
DPC4 gene, 150
dronabinol (Marinol), 104
drug: resistance, 128; side effects, 48, 95

durable power of attorney for health care, 67
DVT (deep vein thrombosis), 100
dying, process of, 61

Engquist, Anna, 23–24, 52, 53
enteral stents, 109–110
EORTC study, 153
epidermal growth factor receptor type 1 (HER1/EGFR), 41
erlotinib, 41, 42f, 153
ESPAC-1 trial, 151, 152t, 153
ESPAC-3 trial, 152
ESPAC-4 trial, 153
evidence-based medicine, 39
executor, choosing an, 52

5-fluorouracil (5-FU), 40, 43, 129, 132, 154t
family: Beth's, 83–84, 87–88; Michael's, 76–78, 81–83, 85–87, 90
family history of cancer: hereditary considerations, 37, 134–135; need for awareness of, 138
fatigue, 32, 43, 97, 98, 100
FDA (Food and Drug Administration), 40, 41, 105
"feeding the cancer," 103
FFCD-SFRO study, 154
Fine, Robert L., 46
FOLFIRINOX (5-fluorouracil, leucovorin, irinotecan, and oxaliplatin), 43
FOLFOX, 129
Food and Drug Administration (FDA), 40, 41, 105
Fragmin, 101
Francis, Prudence, 71
friends, support of, 91–94

gastric outlet obstruction, 104, 109–112, 111f

gastrointestinal (GI) tract, 109
gemcitabine (Gemzar): clinical benefits of, 40; in combination with other drugs, 41–44; in phase 3 studies, 131–132, 134; as second-line therapy, 129–130; as standard adjuvant therapy, 151–155; as standard therapy for pancreatic cancer, 20, 39
genes: BRCA, 13, 37; categories of (proto-oncogenes and tumor suppressors), 149–150
GERCOR, 155
GI (gastrointestinal) tract, 109
GITSG trial, 153, 154
grief, stages of, 62
Grunebaum, Henry, 119–120
GTX (gemcitabine, Taxotere, Xeloda): Columbia University study results, 25, 46–47, 130; development of, 46; pretreatment evaluation for, 47–49; prolonged use of, 31
Guide to the Great Beyond (Brody), 23, 55

H2 (histamine) blockers, 104
hair loss, 41, 43
health care proxy, 54–56, 67, 143, 158–159n5
"hedgehog" molecular pathway, 133
hematology profile (heme-8), 48
hemoglobin, 48
heparins, 101
hepatic artery, 150
hope: and denial, 63; meaning of, 23; realistic, 68–72
hospice care, 44–45, 56, 112–114; open access, 113–114
How We Die (Nuland), 24, 60

immune checkpoint inhibitors,
135–136
immunotherapy, 135
INR (international normalized
ratio) blood test, 101
intravenous nutrition/parenteral
nutrition, 110, 112
irinotecan, 43, 130

jaundice, 12, 16, 102
Johns Hopkins Hospital, 25–27;
Michael's therapy routine at,
27–31; oncology staff, 29–30
Jones, Rick, 133

kidney (renal) function, 47–48,
97
Kimmel Comprehensive Cancer
Center, 27
Kinland, Leonard, 4, 5
Kodish, Eric, 68
K-ras: mutations, 150; pathway as
area for research, 132–133
Kübler-Ross, Elisabeth, *On Death
and Dying*, 62

Last Lecture, The (Pausch), 122
last will, 51, 52, 54, 67, 143
Le, Dung, 1, 6–8
legal documents. *See* advance
health care directives; health
care proxy; last will
lessons learned: about death, 145–
146; after diagnosis, 142–145;
general, 137–140; about treatment, 140–142; about visitors,
90–91
Life after Life (Moody), 59
liver (hepatic) function, 47–48, 97,
101–102, 110
LMWH (low-molecular-weight
heparin), 101

locally advanced/unresectable
disease, 11, 134, 150, 154–155
Lovenox, 101
low-molecular-weight heparin
(LMWH), 101

malabsorption of nutrients, 104
Marinol (dronabinol), 104
Marriott Waterfront Hotel (Baltimore), 91–92
Mayo Clinic, 26
MD Anderson Cancer Center, 26
MDR (multidrug resistance), 128
megestrol (Megace), 104
meta-analysis, definition of, 43
Michael: and aggressive treatment,
22–25; anger, 63–65; and antidepressants, 98; biopsy, 5–8, 10,
17f; CA19-9 results, 13, 116, 118;
CT scan, 4, 16f; and death, 57–
62, 72–74, 118–124; diagnosis
and goals of treatment, 8, 16–19;
diet, 103–105; effects of chemotherapy, 31–37; entitlement,
sense of, 63; and family history
of cancer, 37; and GTX, 39, 45–49,
127–128; hopes, 68–72; pain, 61–
62; performance status, 45; stress,
37–38; symptoms, 4, 11–13, 15–16;
tasks and goals, 51, 53–54; tensions in marriage, 73
mitomycin, 130
Momma and the Meaning of Life
(Yalom), 121
Moody, Raymond A., 59; *Life after
Life,* 59
multidrug resistance phenotype, 128

nab-paclitaxel, 130
nanoalbumin, 131
National Comprehensive Cancer
Network (NCCN): Practice

perioperative (before or after surgery) therapy, 151
platinum agents, 43, 134–135
port, definition of, 34
portal vein, 106, 107f, 108, 150
Post, Stephen, 68
prognosis: discussing with patient and family, 17, 18, 68–72; and performance status, 44; and eligibility for studies, 134
programmed death-1 (PD-1) antibody, 135
proton pump inhibitors, 105
proto-oncogenes, 149–150
pulmonary embolism (PE), 100

radiation, 8, 99, 114, 151–155
rapid autopsy, 125, 131
ras gene, 149; and *K-ras* mutations, 133, 150; *K-ras* pathway, 132
renal (kidney) function, 47–48, 97
resectable (operable) disease, 150–154
respiratory arrest, 67
response rate, 40, 41, 43; in second-line treatments, 128, 130
retroperitoneum, 12, 14f

scans, CT (computed tomography). *See* CT scans
second-line chemotherapy, 128–130
Shepherdstown, W.V., 1, 92–94
signaling: blocking of, 135; in defective genes, 149–150; pathways (in research), 132–133; in targeted agents, 41, 42f
SMA (superior mesenteric artery), 150
small bowel, 12, 102; obstruction of, 109–112, 111f; and the Whipple operation, 151

SMV (superior mesenteric vein), 150
splenectomy, 151
spouse, role of. *See* Beth
"stable disease," 40
stages of pancreatic cancer, 11, 150
"starving the cancer," 103–104
steatorrhea, 16, 104
stents: biliary, 102–103; enteral, 109–110
steroids, 30, 35, 98, 104
stools, 12, 16, 102, 104
stress, 37–38; relieving of, 91–94
Sun, Henry, 3, 5–6
superior mesenteric artery (SMA), 150
superior mesenteric vein (SMV), 150
surgical resection, 11, 13, 18, 150–151, 154
survival rates, 11, 151
survival times, median, 18; and stage of disease, 11; for resectable disease, 151–155; for unresectable disease, 40, 41, 46, 129
Swayze, Patrick, 118
symptoms: ascites, 106; obstruction in gastrointestinal tract, 109; of pancreatic cancer, 11–13, 15–16; pulmonary embolism, 100; unexplained, 37, 138–139

targeted agent, 20, 41, 136
tasks and goals, importance of having, 53–54
Taxotere, 21, 30, 46
Tempero, Margaret, 46
therapy: perioperative (before or after surgery), 151; postoperative (adjuvant), 151–153, 152f; preoperative (neoadjuvant), 151, 153–154

"Travels with Paula" in *Momma and the Meaning of Life* (Yalom), 121

treatment: choosing a place for, 3, 26; decision to receive, 22, 23–24; importance of early, 22–23; nausea and pain during, 49–50; options, 18, 20–21, 39–40; palliative, 18; process of, 27–31; second opinion on, 3, 22, 44, 141; support during, 48–49; surgical, 150–151

tumor: microenvironment of, research on, 132–133; and suppressor genes, 150

ultrasound examination, 2–4, 7
uncertainty principle, 132
unresectable disease, 134, 150, 153
U.S. News and World Report, 26

vena cava filters, 101
ventilation/perfusion (V/Q) scan, 100
visitors, rules for, 90–91
von Gunten, Charles F., 69
Von Roenn, James H., 69

warfarin (Coumadin), 101
Whipple, Allen Oldfather, 151. *See also* Whipple operation
Whipple operation, 36–37, 122, 151
white blood cells, 27, 31–32, 43, 48, 129
will. *See* last will

Xeloda, 21, 30, 32, 43, 46, 95
XELOX, 129

Yalom, Irvin D., 120–121; *Momma and the Meaning of Life,* 121